# Mastering Mechanical Ventilation

# Principles, Practice and Patient Care

Michael J. Dixon, MD, FCCP

Copyright © 2024 by Michael J. Dixon, MD, FCCP

All rights reserved. No part of this publication may be reproduced, distributed, or transmitted in any form or by any means, including photocopying, recording, or other electronic or mechanical methods, without the prior written permission of the author, except in the case of brief quotations used in critical reviews or scholarly articles.

## Preface

The field of mechanical ventilation is a cornerstone of modern critical care, offering life-saving support for patients with respiratory failure, complex pulmonary diseases, and critical illnesses. Mastering Mechanical Ventilation: Principles, Practice, and Patient Care was born out of my years of clinical practice, research, and teaching in pulmonology and critical care medicine. It is designed to address the evolving complexities of ventilator management while ensuring patient-centered care and safety.

This book provides a comprehensive and structured approach to mastering the principles and practice of mechanical ventilation. It is intended to be a reliable resource for medical professionals at all levels, from medical students and residents to seasoned clinicians, nurses, and respiratory therapists. Whether you are encountering mechanical ventilation for the first time or refining your expertise, this book aims to serve as both a foundational guide and a practical reference.

Key features of this text include:

1. Evidence-Based Insights: Grounded in the latest research and clinical guidelines, the book integrates evidence-based practices with real-world applicability to ensure effective and safe ventilator management.

2. Practical Troubleshooting: Mechanical ventilation can be fraught with challenges. This book offers clear guidance on troubleshooting common and uncommon issues, emphasizing a proactive and systematic approach to problem-solving.

3. Case-Based Learning: Through clinical scenarios and illustrative examples, the text bridges theory and practice, helping readers apply concepts to real-world patient care.

4. Comprehensive Scope: From the basics of ventilator modes and settings to the intricacies of managing complex ventilator-induced complications, this book covers the entire spectrum of mechanical ventilation.

As a pulmonologist and critical care specialist, I have witnessed firsthand the challenges and triumphs of managing patients requiring mechanical ventilation. These experiences have informed the content and structure of this book, emphasizing both the technical mastery of ventilator systems and the art of individualized patient care.

I would like to express my gratitude to my colleagues, mentors, and students who have inspired and challenged me throughout my career. Their insights and questions have been instrumental in shaping the depth and breadth of this text. I am also deeply appreciative of my patients and their families, whose courage and resilience continue to motivate my pursuit of excellence in care.

Finally, I hope this book serves as a valuable companion in your journey to mastering mechanical ventilation. By understanding and optimizing this critical tool, we have the potential to not only save lives but also improve the quality of life for countless patients.

Sincerely,
**Michael J. Dixon, MD, FCCP**
Pulmonologist and Critical Care Specialist
2024

Preface
Table of content
List of Abbreviations

## Table of contents

**Chapter One: Fundamentals of Mechanical Ventilation**
- Respiratory Physiology and Mechanics
- Indications for Mechanical Ventilation
- Ventilator Types and Modes

**Chapter Two: Setting Up the Ventilator**
- Initial Patient Assessment
- Key Parameters: Tidal Volume, PEEP, $FiO_2$, and Rate
- Circuit Setup and Alarms

**Chapter Three: Ventilation Strategies for Specific Conditions**
- Acute Respiratory Distress Syndrome (ARDS)

- Chronic Obstructive Pulmonary Disease (COPD)
- Neuromuscular Disorders and Other Conditions

**Chapter Four: Monitoring and Troubleshooting**
- Waveform Analysis and Interpretation
- Identifying and Resolving Common Alarms
- Optimizing Ventilation Parameters

**Chapter Five: Weaning and Extubation**
- Criteria for Weaning Readiness
- Methods of Ventilator Weaning
- Post-Extubation Care

**Chapter Six: Noninvasive Ventilation (NIV)**
- Principles and Applications of NIV
- Patient Selection and Mask Interfaces
- Managing Challenges and Complications

**Chapter Seven: Complications of Mechanical Ventilation**

- Ventilator-Associated Pneumonia (VAP)
- Barotrauma and Volutrauma
- Hemodynamic and Other Systemic Effects

**Chapter Eight: Advanced Topics in Ventilator Management**
- High-Frequency Oscillatory Ventilation (HFOV)
- Extracorporeal Membrane Oxygenation (ECMO)
- Ethical and Palliative Considerations

List of Abbreviations

**ABG**: Arterial Blood Gas

**AC**: Assist-Control Ventilation

**ARDS**: Acute Respiratory Distress Syndrome

**BiPAP**: Bilevel Positive Airway Pressure

**COPD**: Chronic Obstructive Pulmonary Disease

**CPAP**: Continuous Positive Airway Pressure

**ECMO**: Extracorporeal Membrane Oxygenation

**ETCO2**: End-Tidal Carbon Dioxide

**FiO2**: Fraction of Inspired Oxygen

**HFOV**: High-Frequency Oscillatory Ventilation

**ICU**: Intensive Care Unit

**IPPV**: Intermittent Positive Pressure Ventilation

**MV**: Mechanical Ventilation

**NIV**: Noninvasive Ventilation

**PAV**: Proportional Assist Ventilation

**PCV**: Pressure-Controlled Ventilation

**PEEP**: Positive End-Expiratory Pressure

**PIP**: Peak Inspiratory Pressure

**PSV**: Pressure Support Ventilation

**RR**: Respiratory Rate

**SpO2**: Peripheral Capillary Oxygen Saturation

**VAP**: Ventilator-Associated Pneumonia

**VCV**: Volume-Controlled Ventilation

**VT**: Tidal Volume

# Chapter One
# Structure and Function

This chapter begins with an exploration of the critical anatomical structures essential for understanding mechanical ventilation, followed by a review of their physiological functions. The respiratory system, when simplified, can be categorized into two main components: the gas conduction system and the gas exchange system.

Gas Conduction System

The gas conduction system comprises the hollow airways responsible for transporting air to and from the gas exchange system. Beginning at the vocal cords as the trachea, it branches extensively, resembling a tree, until it reaches the acini.

Tracheal and Airway Structure:

The trachea, supported by cartilage and connective tissues, is robust and maintains airway patency.

Progressively, as the airways branch (approximately 16 divisions), they become narrower, lose their cartilage, and exhibit reduced structural support.

Small Airway Vulnerability:

To accommodate millions of acini within the limited thoracic space, smaller airways lack supportive tissues, making them fragile and susceptible to collapse.

Unlike larger airways, which are held open by cartilage and muscle, these smaller passages depend on tension exerted by surrounding tissues for patency.

Factors Influencing Small Airway Diameter:

1. Lung Expansion: Full lung inflation stretches tissues and opens small airways. During exhalation, as tissues relax, airway support diminishes, increasing the risk of collapse.

2. Tissue Properties: Conditions such as emphysema, characterized by loose surrounding tissues, reduce airway stability compared to normal, taut tissues.

Numerosity and Surface Area:

As the tracheobronchial tree branches, the number of small airways increases exponentially, leading to a significant cumulative surface area.

This expanded surface area slows airflow, allowing gas exchange at the acini level to depend on diffusion rather than convection, akin to the gradual tapering of a trumpet.

The increased surface area also minimizes resistance to airflow, ensuring efficient ventilation.

Gas Exchange System

The gas exchange system comprises the acini, alveoli, and the surrounding vascular network. Located at the distal end of the conduction system, this system facilitates the exchange of oxygen and carbon dioxide.

Anatomical Arrangement:

The alveoli, organized into clusters termed acini, create an extensive surface area for gas exchange.

Thin epithelial layers, supported by a basement membrane and capillary endothelium, allow close proximity between alveolar air and blood.

Gas Exchange Mechanism:

Diffusion drives the exchange, governed by concentration gradients. Oxygen moves from higher concentrations in alveolar air to blood, while carbon dioxide follows the reverse path.

Efficient gas exchange requires the maintenance of these gradients, achieved through continuous ventilation.

Ventilation

Ventilation ensures the removal of exhaust gases and replenishment with fresh air, sustaining the necessary concentration gradients for gas exchange.

## Mechanics of Breathing:

## Static Lung Volumes and Pulmonary Mechanics:

At rest, the lung and chest wall settle at the functional residual capacity (FRC), a balance between the lung's inward elastic recoil and the chest wall's outward expansion.

A vacuum in the pleural cavity ensures the lung and chest wall move synchronously.

## Inhalation:

Negative intrathoracic pressure is generated by chest expansion and diaphragm flattening, drawing air into the lungs.

## Exhalation:

Typically passive, exhalation occurs as the diaphragm and chest muscles relax, allowing stored elastic energy and abdominal pressure to expel air.

Forces Influencing Ventilation

Elasticity of the Lung:

Lung elasticity arises from its microarchitecture, similar to the weave of a nylon stocking, and surface tension within the alveoli.

Diseases such as emphysema reduce elasticity by damaging this microarchitecture, while conditions like fibrosis increase stiffness.

Extrathoracic Forces:

Abdominal pressure, as seen in ascites or pregnancy, and external forces, such as chest binders, contribute to exhalation.

Conversely, the outward recoil of the thoracic cage prevents complete airway collapse during exhalation.

Airway Resistance

Airway Diameter:

Resistance to airflow is inversely proportional to the fourth power of airway radius. Large airways (up to the 7th division) contribute most to resistance under normal conditions.

Conditions such as tracheal strictures or the use of small-diameter endotracheal tubes (ETTs) can exacerbate resistance.

Although small airways typically have minimal resistance due to their combined surface area, inflammation or narrowing can rapidly increase resistance, particularly in diseases like bronchiolitis.

Lung Volume and Respiratory Phase as Determinants of Airway Resistance

Lung Volume's Role in Small Airway Diameter

Small airways lack intrinsic structural support and rely on surrounding tissues to remain open. Their diameter is influenced by the degree of tension and stretch in these tissues, which is directly proportional to lung volume. When the lungs are expanded (higher lung volume), the surrounding tissues are taut, pulling the small airways open. Conversely, at lower lung volumes, the surrounding tissue tension decreases, narrowing the airways.

Variation of Resistance During Inhalation and Exhalation

Inhalation, characterized by negative pleural pressures during normal breathing, helps to open small airways. During exhalation, pleural pressures become less negative and may even turn positive in certain regions, reducing the extent to which airways are held open. In severe cases, such as in emphysema, positive pleural pressures may cause airway collapse, particularly when structural support is compromised.

Alveolar pressure during exhalation is higher than atmospheric pressure, which helps to keep the airways open as air exits the alveoli. However, as gas flows through the airways, the pressure diminishes. If this pressure equals the pleural pressure, airway collapse can occur. This balance point, known as the "closing pressure," depends on pleural pressure magnitude and airway narrowing.

Regional Differences in Pleural Pressure

Pleural pressure is not uniform throughout the chest. The weight of the lung and its shape relative to the chest wall create regional variations. For instance, pleural pressures at the lung bases are typically higher due to gravitational effects and the larger lung volume in these areas. Conditions like obesity or emphysema exacerbate these variations, increasing the likelihood of airway closure in regions with higher pleural pressures.

This variability means that even during uniform exhalation, different lung segments may have distinct expiratory flow rates. Some segments may experience obstruction while others remain patent, contributing to ventilation-perfusion (V/Q) mismatches.

Active Exhalation and Forced Expiratory Flow

In individuals with heightened respiratory drive, exhalation can become an active process, facilitated by abdominal muscle contraction. However, increasing thoracic pressure during active exhalation not only propels air out but also compresses small airways. At a critical pressure, airway compression limits the speed of exhalation. This phenomenon is particularly prominent in conditions with reduced airway tethering, such as emphysema.

Forced expiratory flow tests, part of pulmonary function testing, graph the relationship between flow and lung volume. The resulting flow-volume loop illustrates how airway compression during forced exhalation limits airflow. In obstructive lung diseases like emphysema, flow limitations are evident across lung volumes, reflecting severe airway narrowing.

Prolonged Exhalation and Auto-PEEP

In obstructive diseases, exhalation time is significantly prolonged due to increased airway resistance and diminished elastic recoil. When exhalation time exceeds the available respiratory cycle duration, incomplete exhalation leads to gas trapping and dynamic hyperinflation. This phenomenon generates intrinsic positive end-expiratory pressure (auto-PEEP), which exacerbates respiratory effort and fatigue.

Auto-PEEP initially occurs during exertion but may manifest at rest in advanced disease stages. While the increased lung volume from gas trapping enhances airway patency, it also places respiratory muscles at a mechanical disadvantage, further impairing ventilation.

Impact of Lung Disease on Exhalation Mechanics

Diseases affecting lung elasticity or airway resistance alter exhalation dynamics. Emphysema, which erodes elastic recoil, reduces the force driving exhalation while increasing resistance, greatly prolonged exhalation time. Conversely, fibrotic lung diseases enhance elastic recoil, shortening exhalation time. Understanding these dynamics is crucial in managing mechanical ventilation, particularly to prevent auto-PEEP and optimize gas exchange.

Gas Exchange: Oxygen and Carbon Dioxide

## Oxygen Diffusion Dynamics

Oxygen travels to alveolar capillaries primarily by diffusion. In normal lungs, diffusion is rapid and efficient, allowing red blood cells to achieve near-complete oxygen saturation within 0.25 seconds—well within their 0.75-second capillary transit time. However, conditions like thickened alveolar membranes or rapid blood flow (e.g., during exertion) can impair oxygen diffusion, potentially causing hypoxemia. This diffusion impairment is more impactful in diseases with significant alveolar membrane thickening.

## Ventilation-Perfusion (V/Q) Matching

Optimal gas exchange depends on a balanced V/Q ratio. Alveoli with adequate ventilation and perfusion enable efficient oxygen uptake and carbon dioxide elimination. When ventilation exceeds perfusion, excess ventilation does not increase oxygenation beyond saturation limits, representing wasted ventilation. Conversely, insufficient ventilation relative to perfusion leads to hypoxemia. The V/Q ratio across the normal lung averages around 0.8 but varies regionally due to gravity and airway mechanics.

The alveolar gas equation formalizes the relationship between oxygen delivery and removal:

$$PAO_2 = FIO_2 (P_{atm} - 47 \text{ mmHg}) - PaCO_2/R$$

Clinical Implications

1. Obstructive Lung Diseases: Prolonged exhalation times, dynamic hyperinflation, and V/Q mismatch are hallmarks of conditions like asthma and emphysema. Pulmonary function testing, particularly flow-volume loops, aids in diagnosis and monitoring.

2. Restrictive Lung Diseases: Increased elastic recoil in fibrotic diseases shortens exhalation times but reduces lung compliance.

3. Mechanical Ventilation: Understanding auto-PEEP and exhalation dynamics is critical in ventilator management, especially to avoid overdistension and respiratory muscle fatigue.

Diffusion of Carbon Dioxide ($CO_2$)

The diffusion of $CO_2$ from the blood into the alveoli follows a reverse path compared to oxygen. $CO_2$, being more soluble than oxygen, experiences fewer barriers during diffusion. This characteristic makes $CO_2$ diffusion more robust against diseases that disrupt the alveolar membrane.

Ventilation-Perfusion (V/Q) Ratio and $CO_2$ Removal

$CO_2$ removal, like oxygen exchange, relies on the V/Q ratio, though the direction of exchange is reversed. $CO_2$ is transported to the alveoli via the blood, diffuses into the alveolar spaces, and is subsequently exhaled through the airways.

The efficiency of $CO_2$ removal depends on pulmonary ventilation. A well-ventilated pulmonary segment creates a steep diffusion gradient, enhancing $CO_2$ elimination. Conversely, blood flow and the $CO_2$ content within the blood determine the delivery of $CO_2$ to the alveoli.

Low V/Q Ratio

In segments where ventilation is inadequate relative to perfusion (low V/Q ratio), the partial pressure of $CO_2$ ($PaCO_2$) rises. Poorly ventilated acini approach $CO_2$ levels similar to those of the pulmonary arterial blood, limiting the diffusion gradient. Consequently, gas exchange halts once equilibrium is achieved, leaving blood exiting the segment with elevated $CO_2$ levels.

An analogy often used involves a bathtub: the inflow of water represents $CO_2$ delivered from the pulmonary artery, while drainage corresponds to ventilation. Balancing the inflow and outflow is essential to maintain appropriate "water" ($CO_2$) levels.

High V/Q Ratio

In contrast, alveoli with high ventilation relative to perfusion (high V/Q ratio) have lower $CO_2$ concentrations, approaching atmospheric levels. Unlike oxygen exchange, high V/Q ratios do not reach a functional limit for $CO_2$ removal, as ventilation continues to lower acinar $CO_2$ levels, maintaining a favorable gradient for $CO_2$ diffusion.

Compensation by High V/Q Ratio Segments

High V/Q segments can compensate for low V/Q segments by efficiently removing excess $CO_2$ from blood entering the pulmonary veins. This compensatory mechanism provides resilience against V/Q mismatches, helping to stabilize $CO_2$ levels despite impaired ventilation in certain lung areas.

Regulation of Breathing

The brainstem governs respiratory function by integrating signals from sensory inputs, including blood pH, $CO_2$, $O_2$ levels, and mechanical stimuli from the lungs and chest wall. Psychological factors such as anxiety, pain, and fear also influence respiratory control.

The primary driver of respiratory regulation is $CO_2$, due to its critical role in maintaining acid-base balance (pH). Although $O_2$ levels are also monitored, they have a less significant influence, as demonstrated in shallow water blackout scenarios.

To maintain a stable pH, ventilation adjusts to match $CO_2$ production. Elevated $CO_2$ levels trigger increased respiratory rate and depth, often causing discomfort or "air hunger" in individuals unaccustomed to hypercapnia. However, external factors—such as pain, hormonal changes (e.g., in pregnancy or cirrhosis), hypoxemia, and chest pain—can override this respiratory control mechanism.

## Chapter Two
## Respiratory Failure

Understanding the Concept of Failure

Before delving into respiratory failure, it is essential to define "failure" within the context of organ systems. Organ failure occurs when an organ cannot perform the required work to meet specific demands. A useful analogy is that of a tractor towing a trailer. The tractor represents the organ, and the trailer symbolizes the load. Even a healthy tractor can fail if the load is excessive, while a weaker tractor can still function effectively if the load is light.

Similarly, organ failure refers to an organ's inability to meet functional demands. For instance:

Heart failure is the inability to generate sufficient cardiac output without overloading the lungs.

Renal failure is the failure to clear an adequate solute or electrolyte load.

Respiratory failure occurs when the respiratory system fails to provide adequate oxygenation or ventilation.

Respiratory failure is classified into two main types: hypoxemic failure and hypercapnic failure.

Hypoxemic Respiratory Failure

Hypoxemic failure refers to the inability of the respiratory system to achieve sufficient arterial oxygen saturation. Normally, the respiratory system compensates for increased oxygen demand through enhanced cardiac output, which can deliver up to 10 times the resting oxygen supply. However, hypoxemia arises when compensatory mechanisms are overwhelmed.

Causes of Hypoxemic Failure

1. Ventilation-Perfusion (V/Q) Mismatch and Shunts

A V/Q mismatch occurs when the balance between oxygen delivery and blood flow is disrupted.

A shunt represents an extreme V/Q mismatch, where blood bypasses the lungs or where alveoli are perfused but not ventilated.

Common causes include pulmonary embolism, pneumonia, and acute respiratory distress syndrome (ARDS).

2. Diffusion Limitations

Normally, oxygen efficiently diffuses from alveoli to capillaries. However, certain conditions—such as interstitial lung diseases, alveolar filling processes, or pulmonary arterial hypertension—can impair this process, especially during high cardiac output states.

Examples and Mechanisms

Pulmonary Embolism: A blood clot blocks pulmonary arteries, creating "dead space" where ventilation occurs without perfusion. Blood redirected to other lung regions becomes hypoxic due to reduced V/Q ratios.

Pneumonia and ARDS: Alveoli filled with pus or debris cannot participate in gas exchange, creating shunt regions with zero V/Q ratios. Surrounding areas also suffer from reduced ventilation due to inflammation and surfactant loss.

Hypercapnic Respiratory Failure

Hypercapnic failure, also termed ventilatory failure, is characterized by inadequate ventilation to remove carbon dioxide (CO2). While hypoxemia can often be managed with supplemental oxygen, hypercapnia requires direct improvements in ventilation.

Mechanisms of Hypercapnic Failure

Hypercapnia results from an imbalance between CO2 production and removal:

1. CO2 Production

CO2 is generated by metabolism and transported to the lungs for exhalation. Factors increasing CO2 production include:

Fever, vigorous activity, or a carbohydrate-rich diet.

Pathological states like malignant hyperthermia or drug-induced agitation.

2. CO2 Removal

Insufficient ventilation, whether due to reduced respiratory drive or physical barriers to effective breathing, leads to CO2 accumulation.

Key Features of Ventilatory Failure

CO2 accumulation is the hallmark of ventilatory failure.

Factors contributing to inadequate ventilation include neuromuscular weakness, chest wall abnormalities, and reduced respiratory drive.

Summary

1. Hypoxemic Respiratory Failure: Most commonly results from V/Q mismatches or shunting. While diffusion limitations are rare, they may occur in diseases affecting alveolar membranes or pulmonary vasculature.

2. Hypercapnic Respiratory Failure: Arises from insufficient ventilation relative to metabolic demands, with CO2 accumulation being its defining feature.

3. Compensatory Mechanisms: Hypoxic vasoconstriction helps direct blood flow to well-ventilated lung regions, mitigating the effects of hypoxemia in many cases. However, this mechanism can be overwhelmed in severe disease states such as ARDS or pneumonia.

Amount of $CO_2$ Removed per Breath: Revisiting Dead Space

Dead space refers to the volume of air within the respiratory system that does not participate in gas exchange. This includes both anatomical dead space (conducting airways) and alveolar dead space. Dead space ventilation is inefficient as it contributes to overall ventilation without aiding in $CO_2$ elimination. The higher the proportion of dead space, the greater the ventilation required from the functional areas of the lung to maintain normal $CO_2$ clearance.

For example, a patient with zero dead space ventilating at 5 L/min can effectively remove $CO_2$. However, if the same patient has 1 L of dead space, their ventilation rate must increase to 6 L/min to achieve similar $CO_2$ removal, as only alveolar ventilation contributes to gas exchange.

Dead Space and Breadth Depth

The percentage of dead space in a breath depends on its depth. For instance:

With an anatomical dead space of 100 cc, a shallow breath of 200 cc results in 50% dead space, as only 100 cc of air participates in gas exchange.

In contrast, a deep breath of 500 cc reduces the dead space percentage to 20%, leaving 400 cc available for gas exchange.

This demonstrates that shallow breathing requires significantly more ventilation to clear the same amount of $CO_2$ as deeper breathing. Minute ventilation efficiency decreases as dead space fraction increases.

V/Q Mismatch in $CO_2$ Removal

Ventilation-perfusion (V/Q) mismatch also impacts $CO_2$ clearance. While high V/Q segments can compensate for low V/Q segments, significant mismatches may impair $CO_2$ removal, although this is less critical than its impact on oxygenation. Hypercapnia often arises when high V/Q segments are either insufficient in number or entirely absent, as seen in scenarios such as overdoses causing global hypoventilation.

Causes of Ventilatory Failure

1. Respiratory Control System Failure

Inadequate Respiratory Drive
The brain stem normally generates a robust respiratory drive in response to rising $CO_2$ levels. Factors that suppress this drive include:

Drugs: Opioids and benzodiazepines reduce the sensitivity of respiratory centers.

Neurological Events: Increased intracranial pressure or decreased cerebral perfusion can blunt the respiratory response.

Alkalosis: Elevated blood pH, as in hyperventilation-induced shallow water drowning, can suppress respiratory drive.

Case Example: A hyperventilating swimmer induces respiratory alkalosis, then dives and becomes hypoxic without the respiratory drive reactivating before loss of consciousness.

2. Pump Failure (Mechanical Limitation)

Increased Work of Breathing
Conditions like airway obstruction (e.g., asthma, COPD, tracheal stenosis) increase resistance and the effort required to move air.

Obstructive Lung Disease: Small airway collapse during exhalation, exacerbated by diseases like emphysema, narrows the airways, leading to air trapping and hyperinflation.

Restricted Lung or Chest Wall Movement: Pulmonary fibrosis stiffens lungs, while skeletal abnormalities (e.g., kyphosis) reduce chest expansion and diaphragmatic efficiency.

Case Example: A patient with pulmonary fibrosis and kyphosis develops pneumonia, further reducing lung compliance. This combined impairment leads to ventilatory failure.

3. Neuromuscular Limitations

Diseases such as Guillain-Barré Syndrome weaken respiratory muscles, impeding adequate ventilation.

Case Example: A Guillain-Barré patient progressively loses diaphragmatic function, requiring mechanical ventilation.

4. Cardiovascular Limitations

Ventilation depends on sufficient oxygen delivery by the cardiovascular system. Conditions like cardiomyopathy or sepsis can reduce cardiac output, limiting oxygen supply to respiratory muscles.

Acute vs. Chronic Ventilatory Failure

## Chronic Ventilatory Failure

Patients adapt to prolonged high $CO_2$ levels via renal compensation, maintaining normal pH through bicarbonate production. These patients operate near their ventilatory limit, making them vulnerable to acute stressors.

## Acute Ventilatory Failure

Occurs too rapidly for compensatory mechanisms to respond. It can develop independently or as an overlay on chronic failure, where even minor stressors can precipitate acute decompensation.

## Integrated Clinical Perspective

Ventilatory failure results from an imbalance between ventilatory capacity and demand. While healthy individuals have significant reserves, patients with pre-existing limitations (e.g., lung disease, skeletal deformities, or cardiovascular insufficiency) can rapidly progress to failure under increased metabolic demand, such as fever or infection. Management requires addressing both the underlying causes and acute exacerbations to restore ventilatory balance effectively.

## Chapter Three
## Fundamentals of Mechanical Ventilation

Definition of Mechanical Ventilation

Mechanical ventilation is a life-support intervention that utilizes a machine to deliver "mechanical breaths" to ensure proper oxygenation and ventilation of the lungs. The most prevalent type, positive pressure ventilation, operates by pushing air into the patient's lungs, similar to inflating a balloon. This mechanism generates higher-than-atmospheric pressure to drive airflow into the chest.

Conversely, negative pressure ventilators create a vacuum around the patient's thorax, causing chest expansion and air influx due to the pressure gradient. These devices, such as the cuirass or iron lung, are rarely used in intensive care units (ICUs) today and have limited contemporary applications.

Components of a Mechanical Ventilator

At its core, a mechanical ventilator functions as an air pump. While basic ventilators can be manually operated, modern devices incorporate advanced automation, safety features, gas conditioning, and monitoring systems.

Mechanical ventilators typically consist of three primary components:

1. User Interface: This may include a touchscreen or mechanical controls such as knobs and buttons, allowing healthcare providers to interact with the machine.

2. Body: The central unit houses gas mixers, filters, compressors, and pressure adjustment systems. It manages gas intake, conditioning, and output.

3. Ventilator Circuit: Flexible tubing connecting the ventilator to the patient, facilitating the delivery and return of gases.

The ventilator screen prominently displays real-time data, graphical information, and alarms. It also serves as the primary interface for monitoring and controlling the machine.

Ventilator Circuit

The ventilator circuit is a system of tubes through which gas flows between the machine and the patient. Depending on configuration, circuits are classified as:

Dual-limb circuits: Separate tubes for inhalation (inspiratory limb) and exhalation (expiratory limb), commonly used in ICUs.

Single-limb circuits: A single tube for both inhalation and exhalation, with expelled gases vented externally.

In dual-limb systems, a Y-shaped connector joins the inspiratory and expiratory limbs before attaching to the patient's airway via an endotracheal tube, tracheostomy tube, or sealed face mask. Additional devices such as humidifiers, filters, and nebulizers may be integrated to condition the gas and optimize therapy.

Gas Flow and Pressure Regulation

Valves within the ventilator regulate gas flow into and out of the circuit:

Inhalation valves control airflow rates during inspiration.

Exhalation valves modulate gas outflow during expiration.

Sensors positioned within the ventilator or along the circuit measure parameters like pressure and flow, ensuring precise delivery and patient safety.

Pressure and Volume: Core Concepts

Pressure Measurement

Pressure in the ventilator circuit is continuously monitored for safety and therapeutic adjustments. This pressure is influenced by:

Dynamic pressure: Resistance encountered during gas flow through narrow airways or tubing. For example, blowing air through a straw generates dynamic pressure proportional to airflow and airway resistance.

Static pressure: Pressure generated by the elastic recoil of the lungs when they are inflated. It persists even when airflow ceases.

Total pressure is the sum of static and dynamic pressures at any given moment. During the early phase of a mechanical breath, dynamic pressure dominates; as the lungs inflate, static pressure contributes more.

Key Measurements:

1. Peak pressure: The highest pressure recorded during a breath, combining static and dynamic components. A rising peak pressure may indicate airway obstruction, reduced lung compliance, or other issues.

2. Plateau pressure: Measured during a brief pause at the end of inspiration when airflow is stopped. It reflects static pressure alone, providing insights into lung compliance and elasticity.

High plateau pressures suggest reduced lung compliance (e.g., due to pulmonary edema, pneumothorax, or stiff lungs), whereas elevated peak pressures with normal plateau pressures indicate increased airway resistance (e.g., due to mucus plugs or tube kinks).

Volume Measurement

Volume is calculated based on airflow over time. Flow sensors, typically located at the expiratory port, measure gas volume delivered and returned. Discrepancies between administered and returned volumes may signal leaks, tubing disconnections, or other mechanical issues.

Clinical Application and Monitoring

Modern ventilators are equipped to display detailed measurements and alarms, aiding clinicians in optimizing ventilation strategies and promptly addressing complications. Understanding the interplay of pressure, volume, and gas flow dynamics is critical for effective ventilator management, ensuring both patient safety and therapeutic efficacy.

Ventilator Graphics

Modern ventilators are equipped with screens that display various graphics, providing clinicians with a visual representation of ventilator performance. These graphics are invaluable for assessing functionality, troubleshooting alarms, and identifying potential issues. Several key types of ventilator graphics are commonly used:

Pressure-Time Curve

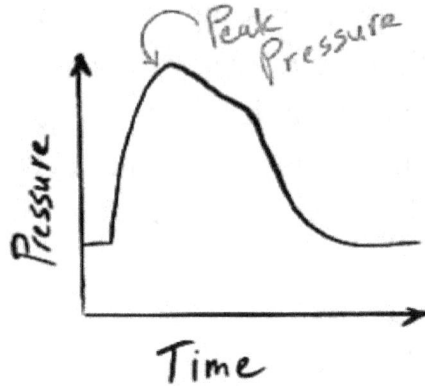

The pressure-time curve illustrates how pressure changes over time during a mechanical breath. This graph offers quick insights into:

Peak Pressure: The maximum pressure achieved during inspiration and when it occurs.

Flow Dyssynchrony: Identifiable as a noticeable dip in pressure before the initiation of the next mechanical breath, which can indicate patient-ventilator mismatch.

54

Work of Breathing: A significant drop in pressure before triggering the ventilator suggests an increased respiratory effort by the patient.

This graphic helps clinicians detect issues such as airflow resistance or inadequate synchronization between the patient and ventilator.

Volume-Time Curve

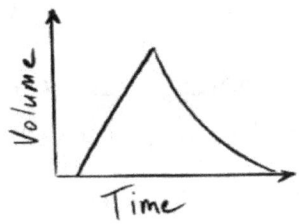

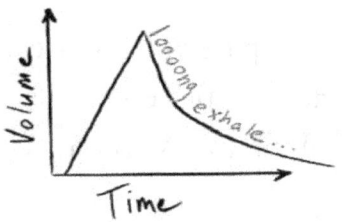

The volume-time curve reflects the amount of air delivered and returned over a specific time frame. It provides insights into:

Delivered and Exhaled Volumes: Monitoring these values ensures that the ventilator is functioning correctly.

Leaks: A discrepancy between inhaled and exhaled volumes may indicate leaks in the ventilator circuit or endotracheal tube.

Gas Infusion: Anomalies in volume trends could point to external sources introducing gas into the system.

This graphic is particularly useful for identifying system leaks, patient disconnections, or unintentional airflow variations.

Ventilator Graphics: Detailed Analysis and Interpretation

Ventilator graphics offer crucial insights into patient-ventilator interaction, enabling clinicians to diagnose, troubleshoot, and optimize care. The following are detailed interpretations of commonly used graphs:

Flow-Time Curve

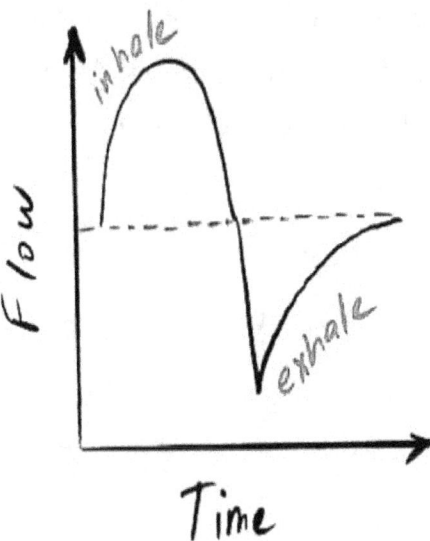

The flow-time curve tracks the rate of gas flow into and out of the patient's lungs over time. Key interpretations include:

Breath Stacking: Overlapping or incomplete exhalations appear as an abnormal flow pattern, indicating improper ventilatory settings.

Gas Infusion Issues: Anomalies in flow patterns may suggest unintended gas introduction from external sources.

Flow Dyssynchrony in Volume-Targeted Breaths: Irregularities in the curve reveal mismatch between the patient's effort and ventilator support.

Volume-Pressure Curve

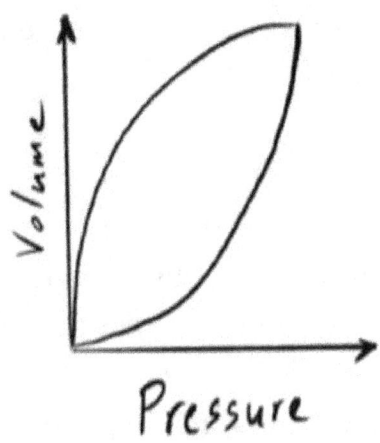

The volume-pressure curve illustrates the relationship between lung volume and airway pressure during ventilation. It provides insights into:

Lung Compliance: A flattened curve or increased slope signifies poor lung compliance, often associated with conditions like ARDS or fibrosis.

PEEP Optimization: A curve that fails to maintain alveolar inflation at end-expiration indicates insufficient positive end-expiratory pressure (PEEP).

Although less precise than static pressure-volume loops obtained during zero flow conditions, the dynamic nature of this graph provides a quick overview of respiratory mechanics and potential compliance changes.

Flow-Volume Loop

The flow-volume loop depicts gas flow relative to lung volume during the respiratory cycle. Its key applications include:

Airway Obstructions: A "scooped" or concave appearance during exhalation suggests obstructive pathologies like COPD.

Treatment Efficacy: Improvements in the loop pattern post-intervention reflect enhanced airway patency.

While not equivalent to forced flow-volume loops used in pulmonary function testing, this graph remains valuable in identifying and monitoring airway resistance trends during mechanical ventilation.

Clinical Relevance

By combining these graphical tools, clinicians can detect ventilation issues such as dyssynchrony, airway resistance, poor lung compliance, or insufficient PEEP settings. Evidence-based analysis of these curves aids in tailoring ventilatory strategies to the patient's unique needs, ensuring optimal respiratory support.

# The Mechanics of Mechanical Ventilation: A Comprehensive Overview

## Understanding the Mechanical Breath

A mechanical breath refers to the inflation of the lungs facilitated by a ventilator. It consists of two phases: inhalation, controlled by the ventilator, and exhalation, which occurs passively without direct ventilator control. Thus, the terms mechanical inhalation and mechanical breath are often used interchangeably. Mastery of this foundational concept is essential for comprehending mechanical ventilation.

## Key Properties of a Mechanical Breath

Three primary properties define a mechanical breath: Target, Time, and Trigger.

1. Target

The target is the specific parameter the ventilator controls, dictating the breath's objective. Common targets include:

Volume Target: Delivers a predetermined volume of gas regardless of airway resistance or lung compliance.

Pressure Target: Maintains a set pressure in the circuit, adjusting the flow dynamically to achieve this goal.

Volume Target Breaths

Mechanism: The ventilator administers a set volume of gas via the inhalation valve. Once the target is reached, the patient exhales through an exhalation port.

Guarantee: Ensures a specific volume is delivered, but circuit pressure varies based on patient factors.

Advantages: Reliable delivery of precise tidal volumes.

Disadvantages: May generate excessive airway pressures, increasing the risk of barotrauma. Fixed flow rates can also lead to patient-ventilator dyssynchrony if they do not match the patient's inspiratory efforts.

Pressure Target Breaths

Mechanism: A driving pressure is maintained by dynamically adjusting gas flow based on feedback from the circuit.

Guarantee: Circuit pressure remains constant, but delivered volumes vary based on lung compliance and patient effort.

Advantages: Reduces the risk of lung injury from high pressures.

Disadvantages: Uncontrolled volumes may result in hypoventilation or excessive inflation if lung compliance changes.

2. Time

The time property determines the duration of inhalation and is controlled by the process of cycling.

Machine-Cycled Breaths: Ventilator stops inhalation based on pre-set parameters such as volume or time.

Volume-Cycled: The breath ends after the target volume is delivered. The flow rate influences delivery speed, with higher rates increasing airway pressures but completing the breath faster.

Flow Patterns:

Square Wave: Delivers gas at a constant flow rate, completing the breath quickly.

Descending Ramp: Gradually reduces flow, simulating natural breathing patterns.

Patient-Cycled Breaths: The patient's effort determines when inhalation ceases.

3. Trigger

The trigger initiates a breath and can be patient-activated (e.g., based on effort) or machine-activated (e.g., time-triggered).

Advanced Targeting: Dual Target Breaths

Dual target breaths integrate both volume and pressure targets, offering the benefits of each mode. For instance, the ventilator adjusts pressure dynamically to achieve a set volume.

Advantages:

Combines precise volume delivery with pressure control to reduce barotrauma risks.

Enhances patient comfort and synchrony in most clinical scenarios.

Disadvantages:

In patients with air hunger, the ventilator may reduce support in response to high initial volumes, increasing patient workload.

Excessive inhalation efforts can lead to lung injury.

Clinical Implications

Understanding these mechanical breath properties allows clinicians to tailor ventilator settings based on patient-specific factors such as compliance, airway resistance, and disease pathology. A careful balance between targets, timing, and triggering mechanisms ensures optimal ventilation while minimizing risks like barotrauma or dyssynchrony.

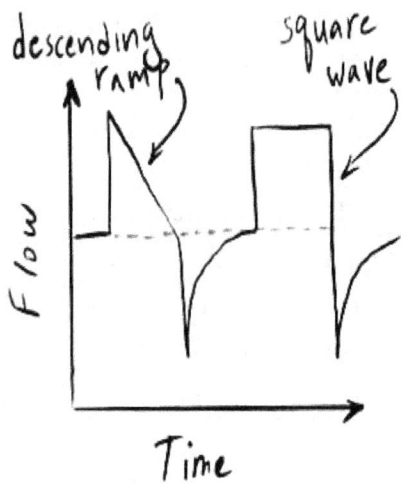

Time-Cycled Ventilation

Definition and Application
Time-cycled ventilation is a mode in which the duration of inhalation is predetermined, ending

automatically when the set time elapses. This mode is commonly associated with pressure-targeted breaths. The inspiratory time (Ti) can be set explicitly or calculated using an inspiratory-to-expiratory (I:E) ratio combined with the respiratory rate. For instance, if the I:E ratio is set to 1:2 and the respiratory rate is 20 breaths per minute, the total cycle time per breath is 3 seconds. Consequently, 1 second is allocated for inhalation and 2 seconds for exhalation.

Advantages

1. Controlled Timing: Ensures precise inhalation durations, which can be tailored to meet clinical needs.

2. Pressure Limitation: Helps avoid overinflation by maintaining the desired pressure within the set time frame.

Limitations

1. Inflexibility: May not accommodate variations in patient effort or changes in lung mechanics, leading to potential discomfort or ventilator dys-synchrony.

2. Dependence on Accurate Settings: Errors in configuring the respiratory rate or I:E ratio can compromise effective ventilation.

Patient-Cycled Ventilation (Flow-Cycled)

Overview
Patient-cycled, or flow-cycled, breaths are terminated based on the patient's respiratory effort rather than fixed parameters. Typically associated with pressure-targeted breaths, these cycles end when the inspiratory flow decreases to a specific threshold, often set as a percentage of the peak inspiratory flow rate (commonly 20%).

## Mechanism

During patient-driven inhalation, gas flows into the ventilator circuit. The flow rate initially rises, reaching a peak, and subsequently declines as the lungs fill. When the flow rate drops to the pre-set threshold (e.g., 20% of the peak inspiratory flow), the ventilator terminates the breath, allowing exhalation.

## Advantages

1. Adaptability: Permits variability in breath duration, accommodating individual patient needs and efforts.

2. Comfort: Aligns with the patient's natural breathing pattern, improving synchrony and reducing discomfort.

3. Feedback on Fatigue: Variations in inspiratory flow patterns can signal patient fatigue or changes in respiratory mechanics, aiding clinical assessment.

## Considerations

1. Operator Expertise: Effective use requires appropriate threshold settings to avoid premature or delayed cycling.

2. Patient Dependence: Relies heavily on patient effort; in cases of weak respiratory drive, it may lead to inadequate support.

## Practical Implications and Case Evidence

### Time-Cycled Scenario
A patient with Acute Respiratory Distress Syndrome (ARDS) may benefit from time-cycled pressure-targeted ventilation. Here, precise control of inspiratory duration ensures optimal alveolar recruitment while minimizing barotrauma.

### Flow-Cycled Scenario
In contrast, a patient recovering from neuromuscular weakness with partial respiratory

effort may find flow-cycled breaths more comfortable. This approach enables the ventilator to adjust breath timing dynamically, reducing the work of breathing and promoting recovery.

Both methods emphasize the importance of aligning ventilator settings with the patient's pathophysiology and comfort to achieve optimal outcomes.

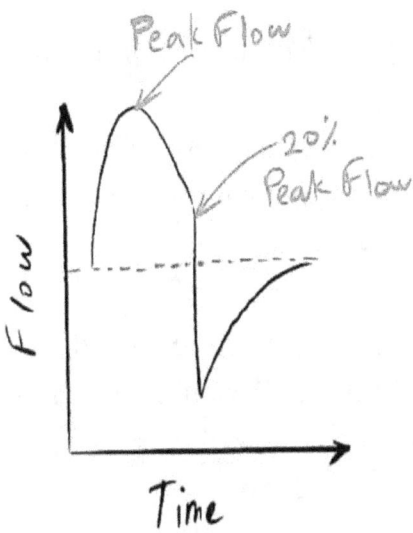

## Understanding Ventilator Triggers and Modes

### Ventilator Triggers

A trigger is the mechanism that initiates a ventilator-delivered breath. Triggers are broadly categorized as either patient-triggered or machine-triggered, depending on whether the patient or the ventilator initiates the breath.

### Types of Triggers

1. Time Trigger (Machine Trigger):

A time trigger relies on a pre-set interval to initiate breaths, ensuring a minimum respiratory rate.

Commonly used in patients who are sedated, paralyzed, or have unreliable respiratory drives, such as those in severe shock.

The ventilator delivers breaths at a fixed rate, regardless of patient effort, serving as a critical backup for maintaining ventilation.

2. Flow Trigger (Patient Trigger):

Activated when the patient inhales, causing a drop in the ventilator circuit's flow.

The ventilator detects this flow change and delivers a breath.

3. Pressure Trigger (Patient Trigger):

Initiated when the patient's inhalation causes a drop in circuit pressure.

Modern ventilators are highly sensitive, minimizing delays and reducing discomfort associated with air hunger.

4. Neurally Adjusted Ventilatory Assist (NAVA):

Less common, this method uses a gastric tube to detect diaphragmatic electrical activity, signaling the need for a breath.

While innovative, this technique is not widely discussed or utilized.

Breath Types

Ventilator-delivered breaths can be classified based on the degree of patient or machine control:

1. Mandatory Breaths:

The ventilator controls at least one aspect, such as the timing or cycling.

Examples:

Time-Cycled, Patient-Triggered Breaths: Initiated by the patient but controlled by the ventilator's timing.

Machine-Cycled, Patient-Triggered Breaths: Initiated by the patient but ended by the ventilator.

2. Spontaneous Breaths:

The patient controls both the initiation and the cycling of the breath.

Typically flow-cycled, allowing for natural variations in breath timing.

3. Assist and Control Breaths (Mandatory Subtypes):

Assist Breaths: Initiated by the patient and delivered with ventilator assistance.

Control Breaths: Fully initiated and cycled by the ventilator.

Ventilator Modes

A ventilator mode determines the combination of triggers, cycling methods, and breath types used during mechanical ventilation.

1. Continuous Mandatory Ventilation (CMV):

Definition: Consists exclusively of mandatory breaths.

Triggering:

Can be time-triggered (by the ventilator) or patient-triggered.

Even patient-initiated breaths are delivered as mandatory breaths, ensuring uniformity.

Targeting Options:

Volume-Control Mode: Delivers breaths targeting a fixed tidal volume.

Pressure-Control Mode: Delivers breaths targeting a specific pressure.

Applications:

Ideal for patients requiring full ventilatory support.

Commonly referred to as "Assist-Control Mode" due to its ability to deliver both assist and control breaths.

2. Modern Advancements in CMV:

Older versions of CMV allowed only control breaths, limiting flexibility. Modern ventilators integrate assist capabilities, enhancing patient-ventilator synchrony.

Clinical Applications

Case Study (Time Trigger):
A sedated ICU patient post-cardiac arrest benefits from CMV with time-triggered breaths, ensuring consistent respiratory support while their neurological status is assessed.

Case Study (Flow Trigger):
A COPD patient on non-invasive ventilation requires a flow trigger to maintain synchrony with the ventilator during spontaneous breathing, reducing air hunger and improving comfort.

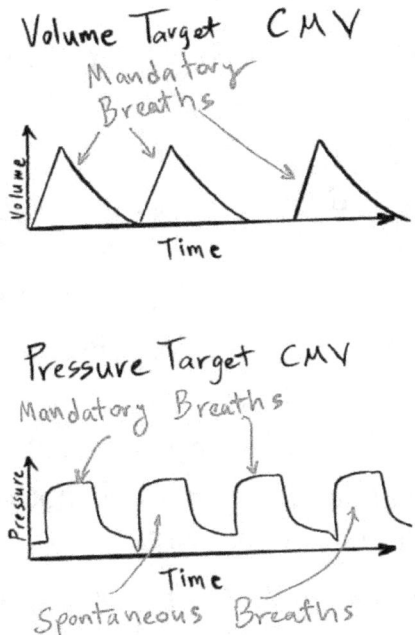

## Intermittent Mandatory Ventilation (IMV)

Intermittent Mandatory Ventilation (IMV) is a ventilatory mode that delivers both machine-triggered and patient-triggered breaths. However, unlike Continuous Mandatory Ventilation (CMV), patient-triggered breaths in IMV are not mandatory. These patient-initiated breaths are either unsupported or categorized as spontaneous, meaning they are both patient-triggered and patient-cycled.

## Synchronized Intermittent Mandatory Ventilation (SIMV)

IMV is often referred to as Synchronized Intermittent Mandatory Ventilation (SIMV) due to its ability to synchronize mandatory and spontaneous breaths. Synchronization ensures that the mandatory breaths do not overlap with patient-initiated breaths. If the ventilator detects that a mandatory breath is due soon, it delivers the mandatory breath even if the patient triggers a breath.

## Clinical Applications and Weaning

Historically, SIMV was commonly used for weaning patients off mechanical ventilation. The machine's mandatory breath rate would be gradually reduced, allowing the patient to transition to spontaneous breathing. However, this approach often prolonged the weaning process and is now largely discouraged in intensive care units (ICUs).

Despite its decline in ICU use, SIMV remains applicable in certain settings:

Long-Term Care Facilities: Slower weaning protocols may still employ SIMV for patients requiring extended ventilatory support.

Neurological ICUs: SIMV can be beneficial for patients with irregular breathing patterns, such as alternating periods of deep, rapid breaths and apnea. The mode ensures a baseline minute ventilation while minimizing dyssynchrony during erratic respiratory patterns.

Key Features of SIMV

Synchronization: Aligns mandatory and spontaneous breaths to avoid overlap.

Flexibility: Accommodates spontaneous breathing while providing ventilatory support as needed.

Specialized Use Cases: Ideal for managing complex respiratory patterns in specific clinical populations.

By understanding its mechanics and limitations, SIMV can be effectively utilized in tailored clinical scenarios, even as its role in routine weaning diminishes.

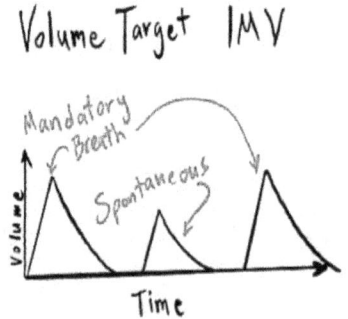

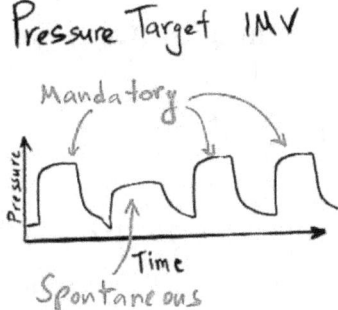

## Continuous Spontaneous Ventilation (CSV)

Continuous Spontaneous Ventilation (CSV) is a ventilatory mode in which all breaths are spontaneous, with no mandatory breaths delivered by the ventilator. This mode allows the patient full control over their respiratory rate and minute ventilation.

## Pressure Support Ventilation (PSV)

When breaths in CSV are pressure-targeted, the mode is often referred to as Pressure Support Ventilation (PSV). This approach is widely utilized as a weaning strategy, particularly in patients transitioning off mechanical ventilation.

Patient Comfort and Safety

CSV is designed to prioritize patient comfort by enabling natural, self-regulated breathing patterns. It is most effective and safe for patients who can maintain consistent and reliable respiratory effort.

Key Features of CSV

No Mandatory Breaths: All breaths are initiated and cycled by the patient.

Autonomy: Patients control both their breathing rate and minute ventilation.

Comfort: Provides a natural breathing experience, ideal for patients ready to assume full respiratory responsibility.

Clinical Application: Commonly used as a weaning mode to facilitate the transition to independent breathing.

CSV represents a patient-centered approach, offering flexibility and comfort while ensuring safe respiratory management in suitable clinical scenarios.

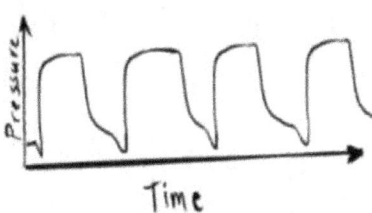

Newer Modes and Techniques in Mechanical Ventilation

Advancements in mechanical ventilation have introduced various modes that go beyond conventional use, offering innovative solutions for specific clinical scenarios. While many of these modes are not yet widely adopted for general patient care, a solid understanding of ventilatory principles provides the foundation for grasping these newer approaches.

Airway Pressure Release Ventilation (APRV)

Airway Pressure Release Ventilation (APRV) is a specialized form of Continuous Spontaneous Ventilation (CSV) with a unique modification. In this mode, the ventilator alternates between two levels of Positive End-Expiratory Pressure (PEEP):

1. High PEEP: This promotes alveolar recruitment, enhancing oxygenation by keeping alveoli open, which is particularly beneficial in conditions associated with hypoxia.

2. Low PEEP: Brief intervals of reduced PEEP allow for effective ventilation and gas exchange.

Spontaneous Breathing Integration

During both high and low PEEP phases, patients retain the ability to breathe spontaneously. This feature is designed to improve comfort and reduce the sense of respiratory dependence by aligning ventilatory support with the patient's natural breathing efforts.

Key Features of APRV

Enhanced Alveolar Recruitment: High PEEP levels aid in maintaining alveolar patency and oxygenation.

Improved Comfort: Spontaneous breathing throughout the cycle reduces ventilator-induced dyssynchrony.

Dual-Level PEEP Cycling: Alternating PEEP levels facilitate both oxygenation and ventilation.

Clinical Applications: Commonly used in cases of acute respiratory distress syndrome (ARDS) and other conditions requiring significant alveolar support.

APRV represents a progressive approach to mechanical ventilation, balancing the benefits of controlled support with patient-driven breathing to enhance outcomes and comfort.

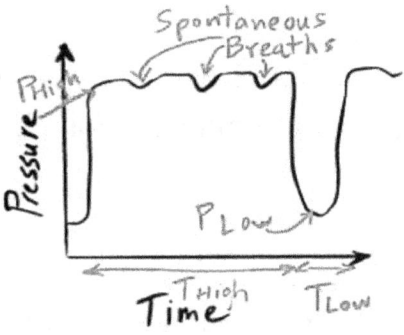

Oxygenation Parameters and Ventilatory Mechanics

Understanding oxygenation parameters and ventilatory mechanics is crucial for optimizing patient care in mechanical ventilation. These settings influence oxygen delivery, exhalation efficiency, and the management of complications such as autoPEEP.

Oxygenation Parameters

Oxygenation parameters are adjustments made to control oxygen delivery within the ventilator's gas mixture and maintain airway pressure between breaths. These include:

1. Fraction of Inspired Oxygen ($FiO_2$):

Adjusted to determine the percentage of oxygen in the gas mixture delivered to the patient.

Typically ranges from 30% to 100%.

2. Positive End-Expiratory Pressure (PEEP):

Represents the pressure maintained in the airway between breaths to prevent alveolar collapse and improve oxygenation.

For detailed guidance, refer to the section on initial ventilator settings.

Exhalation in Mechanical Ventilation

Most ICU ventilators do not enhance exhalation; this phase relies entirely on the patient's respiratory mechanics. Proper exhalation is critical, as physical limitations during this phase can pose significant risks.

Exhalation Mechanics: For a comprehensive understanding, consult the section on respiratory system function.

Exhalation Limitations: Physical constraints during exhalation often result in complications such as autoPEEP (intrinsic PEEP).

AutoPEEP: Definition and Impact

AutoPEEP occurs when insufficient exhalation time prevents the patient from fully exhaling before the next breath begins. This results in progressive gas trapping and increased lung volume, which can cause:

Elevated chest pressure leading to lung overdistension.

Discomfort or pain.

Risk of lung rupture, obstructive shock, or death.

Key Risk Groups:

All mechanically ventilated patients with chronic obstructive pulmonary disease (COPD) experience some degree of autoPEEP.

Patients with airflow obstruction are particularly prone to rapid onset of autoPEEP, even at relatively low respiratory rates.

While small amounts of autoPEEP can be tolerated, excessive buildup can have severe consequences.

Detection and Measurement of AutoPEEP

Recognizing autoPEEP is critical for timely intervention. Common methods include:

1. Clinical Observation:

Listen for continued air flow from the patient at the onset of a new breath.

2. Ventilator Graphics:

Analyze the flow graph. A failure of the flow curve to return to baseline before the next breath may indicate autoPEEP.

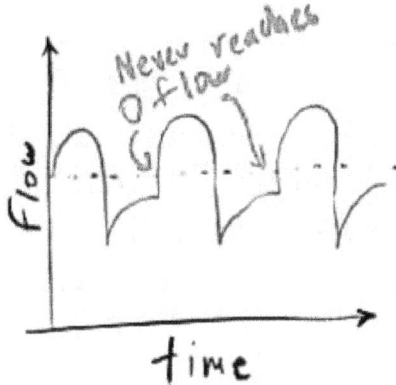

## End-Expiratory Pause and Measuring Intrinsic PEEP

Overview

At the conclusion of exhalation, just before the initiation of a new breath, patients experiencing autoPEEP retain elevated chest pressure above that of the ventilator circuit. This residual pressure is termed intrinsic PEEP, which can be quantified using specific techniques. In normal conditions, without autoPEEP, chest pressure aligns with the circuit pressure, resulting in no airflow.

## Challenges in Measuring Intrinsic PEEP

The ventilator's pressure sensors measure only the circuit pressure, not the internal chest pressure where intrinsic PEEP accumulates. The pressure buildup from autoPEEP occurs in smaller airways beyond the reach of standard sensors.

To illustrate, consider a balloon deflating through a straw:

As long as air flows through the straw, any pressure measurement reflects a value between atmospheric pressure and the balloon's internal pressure.

The true internal pressure of the balloon can only be measured by halting the flow, allowing the pressure within the straw to equilibrate with the balloon's internal pressure.

Similarly, intrinsic PEEP in the lungs must be measured by pausing airflow to achieve equilibrium.

Principle of End-Expiratory Pause

To accurately measure the intrinsic PEEP:

1. Stop Airflow: Just before the next breath, airflow out of the circuit is paused.

2. Pressure Equalization: This pause allows the pressure across the tubing and within the patient's chest to stabilize.

3. Measure Intrinsic PEEP: Once equilibrium is achieved, the pressure reading obtained represents the intrinsic or autoPEEP.

This principle is integral for assessing pressures in otherwise inaccessible spaces and is applicable in other clinical contexts, such as measuring plateau pressure and using Swan-Ganz catheters.

Clinical Relevance

Understanding and utilizing the end-expiratory pause technique is essential for:

Detecting and quantifying autoPEEP.

Preventing complications associated with elevated intrinsic PEEP, such as lung overdistension and hemodynamic compromise.

Ensuring accurate ventilator management in patients with airflow resistance.

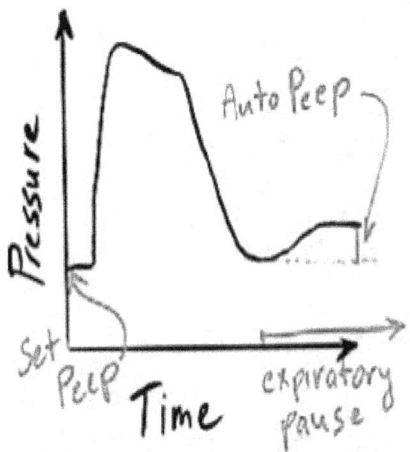

Management of AutoPEEP and Ventilator Dyssynchrony

Immediate Interventions for AutoPEEP

In cases where autoPEEP causes hemodynamic instability or shock, disconnecting the patient from the ventilator allows for immediate decompression and temporary improvement in hemodynamics. However, this is a short-term measure as the issue will recur upon reconnection. A more sustainable solution involves addressing the underlying mismatch between exhalation time and the time required for complete exhalation.

Strategies to Manage AutoPEEP

1. Increasing Exhalation Time

Adjust Inspiratory Flow Rates:
Increasing inspiratory flow rates reduces inhalation time, indirectly extending exhalation time. This can be achieved by increasing maximum inspiratory flow, switching to a square wave flow pattern, or adjusting inspiratory time (Ti).

Limitations: While this method may provide a slight time gain, it often increases dynamic inspiratory pressures. Additionally, patients may inadvertently increase their respiratory rate in response to higher flow rates, limiting its effectiveness.

Reducing Respiratory Rate:
Lowering the respiratory rate provides more time for exhalation. However, this approach can be challenging in patients with high respiratory drive or agitation. Sedation or analgesia may be required, and in extreme cases, paralytics may be used, though only as a last resort and in conjunction with adequate sedation.

2. Reducing Exhalation Time Requirements

Decrease Tidal Volume:
Smaller tidal volumes result in reduced gas volume to exhale, shortening exhalation time. However, this must be balanced against the patient's minute ventilation needs to maintain acid-base balance.

Minimize Airway Resistance:
For large airway obstructions, interventions such as suctioning secretions or using larger endotracheal tubes can help. In cases of bronchiolar resistance, as seen in COPD or

asthma, bronchodilators and corticosteroids can alleviate bronchospasm.

## Ventilator Settings for Optimizing Exhalation

Mechanical ventilators must be carefully configured to ensure adequate exhalation time:

Calculation of Expiratory Time: The time for exhalation is determined by subtracting inspiratory time from the total respiratory cycle duration. For example, a respiratory rate of 10 breaths per minute provides 6 seconds per cycle; if inhalation takes 2 seconds, 4 seconds remain for exhalation.

Avoiding Breath Stacking: Mild breath stacking may function as additional PEEP and is often tolerated, but significant stacking leads to detrimental outcomes, including severe autoPEEP.

Ventilator Dyssynchrony and its Implications

Ventilator dyssynchrony arises from a mismatch between the patient's intrinsic respiratory efforts and ventilator settings. This mismatch can increase mortality, exacerbate lung stress, prolonged mechanical ventilation, and elevate sedation requirements.

Types of Dyssynchrony

1. Failure to Trigger:

Occurs when the patient cannot generate sufficient negative pressure to initiate a breath, often due to autoPEEP or hyperinflation.

Management: Increasing exhalation time, treating airway obstruction, reducing tidal volume or respiratory rate, and optimizing PEEP settings.

2. Flow Dyssynchrony:

Results from inadequate flow delivery during inspiration, leading to patient discomfort.

3. Time Dyssynchrony:

Happens when ventilator breath duration does not align with the patient's effort, resulting in a breath that is too short or too long.

4. Auto-Triggering:

Ventilator delivers unrequested breaths, typically due to circuit leaks or inappropriate sensitivity settings.

Optimizing PEEP for Dyssynchrony and AutoPEEP

Adjusting the PEEP set can help by reducing the pressure difference the patient needs to overcome to trigger the ventilator.

Guidelines for Adjusting PEEP:

Set PEEP to approximately 75% of the estimated intrinsic PEEP.

Increase PEEP gradually and monitor the patient's response closely to avoid exacerbating autoPEEP.

Over-adjusting PEEP may worsen gas trapping and lead to further complications.

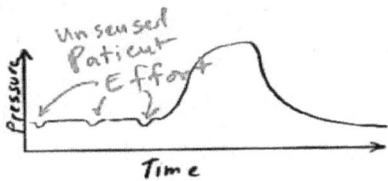

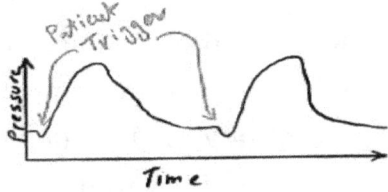

Flow Dyssynchrony: Causes, Impact, and Management

Flow dyssynchrony arises when the ventilator's flow rate fails to meet the patient's breathing demands. This issue is specific to flow-limited modes, such as volume-targeted ventilation, where the flow rate and pattern are preset.

Consequences of Flow Dyssynchrony

Severe flow dyssynchrony can result in "double triggering," where the ventilator delivers two consecutive breaths without allowing for exhalation. This subjects the lungs to double the intended tidal volume, increasing the risk of lung overdistension. Even without double breaths, the patient's effort to compensate creates tension on lung tissues, particularly in the lung bases, which are more prone to localized overdistension due to atelectasis or underlying disease. This disproportionate stress can contribute to pulmonary complications, including edema caused by elevated transmural vascular pressures.

Patients with heightened respiratory drive—due to pain, agitation, acidemia, or anemia—are especially vulnerable to flow dyssynchrony. The mismatch between their inspiratory effort and the ventilator's flow delivery often leads to patient discomfort, agitation, and increased work of breathing.

Pathophysiology of Flow Dyssynchrony

In cases of flow dyssynchrony, the patient inhales gas faster than the ventilator can provide it. This mismatch creates a pressure drop in the circuit. If severe enough, this drop may trigger an additional breath, compounding the issue. The sensation of inadequate airflow exacerbates discomfort, akin to the experience of breathing through a blocked nasal passage.

Approach to Management

Addressing flow dyssynchrony involves interventions targeting both the patient's condition and ventilator settings:

Patient-Focused Interventions

1. Treat Underlying Causes: Address conditions driving the patient's increased respiratory effort, such as acidemia, fever, anemia, or agitation.

2. Symptom Management: Administer appropriate anxiolytics or analgesics to alleviate pain or anxiety contributing to the respiratory drive.

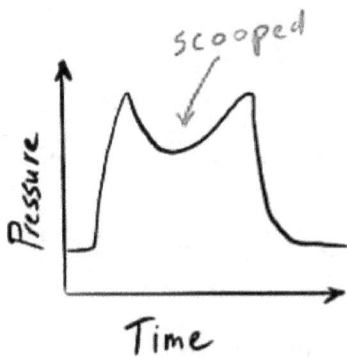

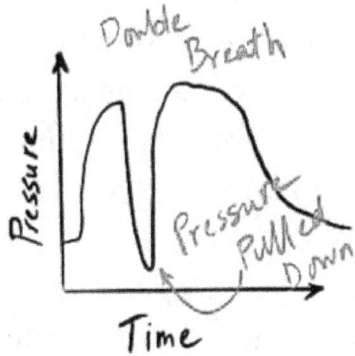

Ventilator Adjustments

1. Increase Flow Rate: Raising the ventilator's flow rate can better match the patient's demand but may shorten breath duration. Care must be taken to avoid premature cycling of the ventilator, which could worsen the dyssynchrony.

2. Modify Flow Patterns: Experiment with different flow waveforms to identify one that aligns with the patient's respiratory pattern.

3. Switch to Pressure-Controlled Modes: In pressure-controlled ventilation, flow is not restricted, allowing patients to take large breaths. However, excessive tidal volumes in this mode may risk lung injury.

4. Consider Dual-Target Modes: While these modes adjust to patient effort, they may inadvertently increase the patient's work of breathing by reducing support pressure.

In cases of severe flow dyssynchrony, temporary adjustments, such as allowing a slightly higher tidal volume, may be warranted until the underlying condition driving the air hunger is addressed.

Time Dyssynchrony: Causes, Identification, and Management

Time dyssynchrony occurs when the duration of a ventilator-delivered breath does not align with the patient's natural respiratory drive. This mismatch can lead to significant mechanical and physiological challenges.

Mechanisms and Implications

1. Breath Too Short:
When the mechanical breath ends prematurely, the patient's continued inspiratory effort may trigger another breath before exhalation occurs. This results in "double triggering" or "double breaths," potentially doubling the tidal volume and increasing the risk of lung injury.

2. Breath Too Long:
Conversely, if the ventilator breath is prolonged, the patient may initiate exhalation while the ventilator is still delivering gas. This leads to elevated airway pressures as the lungs resist further inflation, which may increase the risk of barotrauma or patient discomfort.

Detection via Ventilator Graphics

Ventilator waveforms provide critical insights into time dyssynchrony:

Short Mechanical Breaths:

The flow-time curve may show incomplete or absent flow reversal at the end of inhalation.

The pressure-time curve may display a drop below baseline, occasionally accompanied by double breaths.

Prolonged Mechanical Breaths:

The pressure-time curve shows a spike at the end of the breath, reflecting patient resistance to continued inflation.

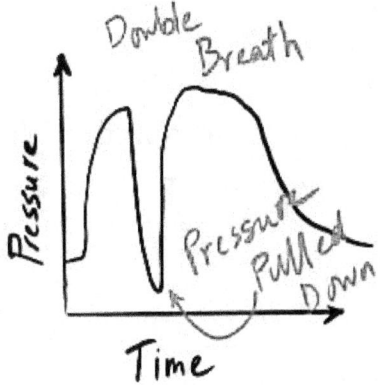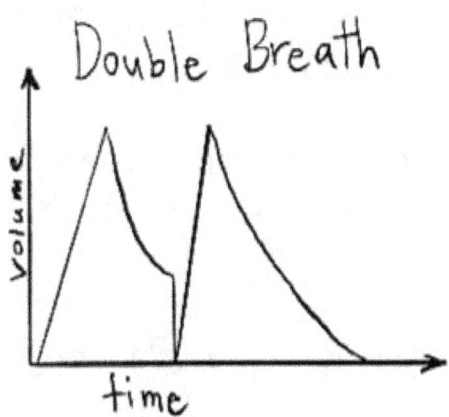

## Management Strategies

Addressing time dyssynchrony involves optimizing ventilator settings and addressing underlying patient factors:

### Ventilator Adjustments

1. Match Breath Duration:

In volume-targeted modes, adjust the flow rate or flow pattern to better align with the patient's inspiratory effort.

In pressure-targeted control modes, modify the inspiratory time (Ti) to match the patient's requirements.

2. Switch to Flow-Cycled Modes:

Spontaneous pressure support modes allow the patient to control the duration of each breath, reducing the risk of dyssynchrony.

Address Patient Factors

Patients experiencing air hunger often demand prolonged inhalations. Identifying and managing the underlying causes of air hunger can alleviate this issue:

Treat acidosis to reduce the drive for deep breaths.

Manage fever, pain, or other conditions contributing to increased respiratory effort.

Autotrigger: Identification, Implications, and Management

Definition and Causes
Auto Triggering occurs when a ventilator delivers a breath without an actual inspiratory effort from the patient. Modern ventilators are highly sensitive, designed to detect minimal changes in flow or pressure to facilitate

comfortable and efficient breathing. However, this sensitivity can inadvertently respond to non-respiratory events, such as:

Hiccups, tremors, or cardiac oscillations caused by vigorous heartbeats.

Circuit leaks, including minor leaks around endotracheal tube cuffs or disconnections in the ventilator circuit.

Clinical Implications

Auto Triggering can lead to over-ventilation, resulting in respiratory alkalosis, characterized by:

Spasms or tetany.

Neurological symptoms, such as seizures.

Cardiac arrhythmias due to altered ionized calcium levels.

## Recognition

Auto Triggering is often identified by:

Ventilator waveforms showing breaths delivered without any visible patient effort.

Clinical suspicion in cases of respiratory alkalosis while the patient is on mechanical ventilation.

## Management

1. Assess Ventilator Settings:

Check and adjust trigger sensitivity to reduce unnecessary breaths while avoiding increased patient effort.

Inspect for leaks in the circuit or around the endotracheal tube.

2. Eliminate External Triggers:

Identify and address external factors such as tremors or cardiac oscillations.

3. Ensure Circuit Integrity:

Verify the placement and cuff integrity of the endotracheal tube.

Check for any disconnection or malfunction in the ventilator setup.

Ventilator Alarms: Types, Causes, and Troubleshooting

Peak Pressure or High Inspiratory Pressure Alarm

This alarm indicates elevated pressure in the circuit, potentially due to:

Obstruction: Patient coughing, kinked tubing, or secretions in the airway.

Reduced Compliance: Pneumothorax, lung edema, or chest wall stiffness.

Action Steps:

Check for kinks or biting on the tubing.

Suction airway secretions.

Perform lung auscultation for symmetrical air entry.

Order imaging, such as a chest X-ray or bedside ultrasound, to rule out pneumothorax or other conditions.

Measure plateau pressure to differentiate between airway resistance and compliance issues.

Leak Alarm

Triggered when the ventilator detects a discrepancy between delivered and returned flow. Common causes include:

Endotracheal tube cuff leaks or migration.

Circuit disconnections or leaks.

Action Steps:

Inspect the circuit for audible or palpable leaks.

Ensure the endotracheal tube is positioned correctly (2-4 cm above the carina).

If significant leaks are present, reposition or replace the endotracheal tube immediately.

Low Pressure Alarm

Indicates a significant drop in circuit pressure, often due to:

Large leaks or circuit disconnections.

Excessive patient effort during exhalation.

Action Steps:

Investigate for circuit disconnections or damaged components.

Ensure the endotracheal tube is secure.

Patient Disconnect Alarm

Triggered by a dramatic drop in resistance and pressure, often signifying:

Accidental disconnection or extubation.

Action Steps:

Immediately reconnect or re-intubate the patient if necessary.

Low Tidal Volume and Low Minute Ventilation Alarms

Indicate insufficient exhaled volume, potentially caused by:

Inadequate ventilator support in pressure-targeted modes.

Patient fatigue during weaning trials.

Premature breath termination in volume-targeted modes due to high-pressure cutoffs.

Action Steps:

Adjust ventilator support or reassess readiness for weaning.

Investigate for underlying causes of high-pressure alarms.

## High Minute Ventilation Alarm

Occurs when measured minute ventilation exceeds set limits, possibly due to:

Patient hyperventilation caused by pain, anxiety, or metabolic acidosis.

Auto Triggering.

Action Steps:

Address underlying causes such as pain or anxiety.

Reassess ventilator sensitivity to prevent auto triggering.

## High Exhaled Tidal Volume Alarm

Indicates an abnormally large exhaled volume, often due to:

Stacked breaths or inadvertent gas flow into the circuit (e.g., from a nebulizer).

Action Steps:

Confirm that no external gas sources are connected to the circuit.

Evaluate the cause of stacked breaths using ventilator waveforms.

## Apnea Alarm

Triggered when a spontaneous breath is not detected within a preset time, common in:

Over-sedation.

Neurological compromise.

Action Steps:

Assess sedation levels and adjust as necessary.

Investigate for neurological changes and manage underlying causes.

## Conclusion

Effective management of ventilator alarms and auto triggering involves understanding their underlying mechanisms, using ventilator waveforms for assessment, and addressing both mechanical and patient-related factors. Quick, systematic troubleshooting ensures patient safety and optimal respiratory support.

## Chapter Four
## Correcting Respiratory Failure

Management of Hypoxemia

Hypoxemia, a critical medical emergency, requires immediate correction as it is poorly tolerated. Fortunately, various interventions exist to address this condition. This chapter outlines passive oxygen supplementation methods, the role of mechanical ventilation, and strategies to address hypercapnia.

1. Oxygen Supplementation: Passive Methods

Supplemental oxygen increases alveolar oxygen pressure, improving oxygen delivery even in poorly ventilated alveoli, and corrects issues stemming from ventilation-perfusion (VQ) mismatch. It can also address oxygenation challenges in alveoli with diffusion defects by creating a steeper diffusion gradient.

However, supplemental oxygen cannot resolve shunt-related hypoxemia, as shunted blood bypasses ventilated alveoli, negating oxygen supplementation benefits.

Delivery Methods

1. Nasal Cannula:

Most common and minimally invasive.

Delivers oxygen at 5 L/min (standard) or up to 10 L/min (high-flow).

Oxygen concentration varies due to entrained room air, which depends on the patient's respiratory rate and inspiratory flow.

High-flow nasal cannulae allow humidification, improving patient comfort.

2. Face Masks:

Offer a higher concentration of oxygen by reducing room air entrainment.

A venturi device can control oxygen concentrations (e.g., 30%–90%) using principles like the Bernoulli effect. However, room air dilution still occurs based on patient-specific needs.

3. Reservoir Devices:

Examples include non-rebreather masks and nasal reservoir systems (e.g., Oxymizer).

Reservoirs provide an initial oxygen-rich gas volume during inhalation, reducing room air entrainment.

These devices are typically used short-term due to their desiccating effects, which can cause discomfort and dry out secretions.

4. High-Flow Oxygen Systems:

Deliver flow rates up to 50 L/min, minimizing room air dilution and ensuring adequate oxygen delivery.

High-flow devices are often humidified for enhanced patient comfort.

Passive oxygen supplementation has limitations. For patients requiring further support, mechanical ventilation becomes necessary.

2. Mechanical Ventilation

Mechanical ventilation introduces positive pressure to inflate the lungs, enhancing oxygenation and resolving hypoxemia. This method eliminates ambient air entrainment, guaranteeing the prescribed oxygen concentration.

## Mechanisms of Action

1. Improved Oxygen Delivery:

Creates a sealed interface, ensuring the delivery of precise oxygen concentrations.

2. Lung Recruitment:

Reopens collapsed alveoli (atelectasis) through positive airway pressure, converting non-functional lung segments into active participants in gas exchange.

Positive End-Expiratory Pressure (PEEP) prevents alveolar collapse between breaths, mitigating atelectrauma.

3. Reduced Oxygen Utilization:

Mechanical ventilation decreases respiratory muscle workload, reducing the metabolic demand for oxygen.

Sedation or paralysis, when required, further minimizes oxygen consumption.

4. Correction of Hypoventilation:

Alleviates the fatigue associated with insufficient ventilation, ensuring adequate oxygenation.

Cautions in Oxygen Therapy

Oxygen, though essential, can cause oxidative stress at high doses. Overuse may lead to absorption atelectasis. Evidence suggests maintaining oxygen saturation at 94%–98% improves outcomes in patients receiving non-invasive oxygen therapy. A similar conservative approach is being evaluated for mechanically ventilated patients.

3. Correction of Hypercapnia

Hypercapnic respiratory failure arises from a mismatch between minute ventilation and the patient's metabolic requirements for carbon dioxide ($CO_2$) clearance. Unlike oxygen, $CO_2$ removal cannot be enhanced by supplementation; mechanical ventilation is the primary intervention.

Mechanical Ventilation Mechanisms

1. Guaranteed Minute Ventilation:

Ensures a consistent level of ventilation in patients with impaired respiratory drive.

2. Augmented Work of Breathing:

Supports or replaces the patient's effort to meet ventilatory demands, preventing respiratory fatigue.

3. Lung Recruitment:

Opens collapsed or poorly ventilated lung segments, improving $CO_2$ clearance.

4. Reduced $CO_2$ Production:

Sedation or paralysis decreases metabolic activity, reducing $CO_2$ production.

Key Considerations

Sedative medications must be used cautiously in non-ventilated patients with hypercapnic failure, as they risk worsening respiratory depression.

Summary

Hypoxemia: Manage conservatively using oxygen supplementation, escalating to mechanical ventilation as needed. Maintain oxygen saturation between 94%–98%.

Hypercapnia: Relies solely on mechanical ventilation to augment $CO_2$ clearance, supported by strategies to decrease metabolic demand and recruit functional lung tissue.

These interventions form the cornerstone of managing respiratory failure in critically ill patients.

## Chapter Five
## Initiating and Setting Mechanical Ventilation

Indications for Mechanical Ventilation

Mechanical ventilation is primarily indicated in cases of respiratory failure, airway protection during surgery, or when the patient exhibits a compromised mental state. However, not all patients in respiratory distress or with altered mental status require mechanical ventilation. The decision to initiate mechanical ventilation is based on a thorough clinical assessment, considering vital signs, laboratory results, disease progression, anticipated therapeutic response, and overall clinical trends.

It is crucial to approach this decision carefully, as mechanical ventilation carries potential risks. Initiating ventilation can lead to hemodynamic instability, potentially precipitating a patient's decompensation. If endotracheal intubation is necessary, the procedure itself introduces further risk. Additionally, mechanical ventilation can increase the likelihood of pneumonia and other complications associated with immobility.

A significant danger is the delay in initiating mechanical ventilation. As a patient's condition deteriorates, the risks of intubation and subsequent complications increase. Once respiratory failure reaches an advanced stage, intubation becomes more challenging, non-invasive ventilation (NIV) becomes less effective, and the potential for post-intubation complications rises.

Airway Protection and Mental Status

Approximately 20% of intensive care unit (ICU) patients are intubated for airway protection. A compromised ability to protect the airway significantly increases the risk of respiratory failure due to apnea, hypoventilation, or aspiration. A key factor in determining airway protection is the Glasgow Coma Scale (GCS). A GCS score below 8 is often used as an indicator for intubation, based on trauma studies that highlight the risks of apnea, aspiration, and hypoventilation in patients with a GCS of 8 or lower. However, the decision must be individualized. For example, patients with vomiting, excessive secretions, or signs of respiratory distress may require intubation even if their GCS is above 8.

It's important to note that the gag reflex is not a reliable indicator of airway protection. Assessing a patient's response to verbal commands provides better insight into their ability to handle secretions. If a patient is unable to manage their secretions effectively or requires maneuvers like jaw thrust to maintain the airway, intubation should be considered, unless the condition is rapidly reversible, such as in cases of opioid overdose.

Respiratory Failure – Hypoxemia

Progressive hypoxemia that requires escalating oxygen supplementation is an indication for intubation, particularly if the patient's oxygen needs exceed the capacity of non-invasive methods. Waiting until hypoxemia becomes severe can complicate the intubation process, as it may lead to rapid desaturation and worsen the difficulty of securing the airway.

High-Risk Patients for Respiratory Failure

Certain patients are particularly vulnerable to sudden respiratory failure due to either catastrophic respiratory muscle failure or a propensity for insidious $CO_2$ accumulation.

Signs of Respiratory Fatigue

Rapid, shallow breathing

Irregular or erratic breathing patterns

Complaints of dyspnea

Diaphoresis (excessive sweating)

Agitation or, more dangerously, somnolence

Tachycardia, hypertension, or arrhythmias

Paradoxical breathing and use of accessory muscles

Shock

Patients in shock, such as those with sepsis or myocardial infarction, are at heightened risk for respiratory arrest due to oxygen deprivation of respiratory muscles. In these cases, early intubation should be considered.

High Work of Breathing

Patients experiencing high work of breathing, such as those with severe asthma or other obstructive conditions, are also at risk for sudden deterioration. These patients may initially manage the increased work but can rapidly worsen and arrest. Monitoring asthmatic patients in status is critical, as signs of fatigue or improvement in CO2 levels may indicate the need for intubation. The decision to intubate is particularly challenging, given the risks associated with intubation in such patients.

Neuromuscular Disease

Patients with neuromuscular diseases are also at significant risk for progressive ventilatory failure. Respiratory arrest can occur suddenly after a prolonged period of silent respiratory insufficiency, especially when these patients are sleeping or less closely monitored. Neuromuscular diseases often present with multiple factors, such as weak respiratory muscles, difficulty clearing secretions, and atelectasis, which contribute to failure.

Close monitoring of respiratory parameters—such as Forced Vital Capacity (FVC), Negative Inspiratory Force (NIF), and Maximal Expiratory Pressure (MEP)—is recommended for these patients. In

Guillain-Barré syndrome (GBS), a "20-30-40" rule can help guide the decision to intubate: an FVC below 20, NIF below -30, or MEP below -40 warrants consideration for intubation. Other signs of respiratory failure in neuromuscular disease include dyspnea, tachypnea, paradoxical breathing, and difficulty speaking in full sentences. Hypoxemia and hypercapnia are late signs, and waiting for these indicators may result in the need for emergency intubation, which carries greater risks.

Invasive vs. Non-Invasive Mechanical Ventilation

Mechanical ventilation can be administered through either an invasive or non-invasive interface, each with distinct advantages and limitations.

Invasive Mechanical Ventilation

Invasive mechanical ventilation involves the use of an endotracheal tube or tracheostomy tube.

The main advantage is that it bypasses the upper airway, ensuring a secure airway and allowing for deep sedation without concern for airway obstruction. This method guarantees the delivery of the prescribed gas mixture and pressure to the lungs. Additionally, it provides protection against large aspiration events due to the inflated cuff and enables effective pulmonary hygiene, such as suctioning.

However, the major drawback is that invasive ventilation bypasses the protective reflexes of the upper airway, increasing the risk of pneumonia and other complications. The procedure itself—intubation—also carries inherent risks, including difficulty in securing the airway.

Non-Invasive Mechanical Ventilation

Non-invasive mechanical ventilation (NIV) utilizes a face mask to deliver ventilatory support, allowing the upper airway's protective mechanisms to remain intact. This method avoids the need for sedation and reduces complications related to airway trauma, making it more comfortable for the patient. However, it is less effective in patients who are unable to maintain airway patency, particularly those with unstable mental status or heavy sedation. NIV also does not provide protection against aspiration.

NIV is most beneficial in patients with chronic obstructive pulmonary disease (COPD) exacerbations, pulmonary edema, or immunocompromised pneumonia, where it has been shown to reduce the need for intubation, shorten hospital stays, and decrease mortality. However, its use in acute hypoxemic failure should be approached cautiously, as failure to intubate in a timely manner may worsen the patient's condition.

Contraindications to Non-Invasive Ventilation

Hemodynamic instability

Inability to protect the airway (GCS < 8)

Excessive secretions

Uncooperative or agitated patients

Recent upper gastrointestinal or airway surgery

Respiratory arrest

## Setting the Pressure Target for Breath Delivery

### Driving Pressure

In pressure-targeted ventilation, the appropriate driving pressure ensures adequate ventilation while minimizing the pressure to which the lungs are exposed. A typical starting point for driving pressure is 20 cm H2O, adjusted to achieve a tidal volume of approximately 6 mL/kg of the patient's ideal body weight. The total pressure the lungs receive is the sum of the driving pressure and positive end-expiratory pressure (PEEP), which should be limited to around 30 cm H2O to prevent excessive lung stress.

Inspiratory Time and I:E Ratio
For a pressure control breath, the inspiratory time and the inspiratory-to-expiratory (I:E) ratio need to be carefully adjusted. The inspiratory time determines how long the driving pressure is applied to the ventilator circuit, while the I:E ratio dictates the proportion of time spent inhaling compared to exhaling. For instance, a patient breathing at 15 breaths per minute has 4 seconds per cycle: 1 second for inspiration and 3 seconds for expiration, giving an I:E ratio of 1:3. Ideally, the I:E ratio should be around 1:2 to mimic normal respiration. Conditions like obstructive diseases may require a longer expiratory phase, and hypoxic patients may benefit from a longer inspiratory phase.

Setting Respiratory Frequency
The respiratory frequency is set based on the target minute ventilation, typically aiming for 5-7 L/min, depending on the patient's needs. In

cases of obstructive lung diseases, longer exhalation times may be required. If the patient is able to initiate their own breaths, they should be allowed to do so unless there is a reason to maintain deep sedation or paralysis. If a patient is not over-breathing, the cause should be investigated, as it could indicate issues such as sedation or over-ventilation.

Oxygenation Settings

Fraction of Inspired Oxygen (FiO2) and PEEP
Upon initiating mechanical ventilation for a critically ill patient, FiO2 is usually set to 100%. This is then gradually titrated down to maintain oxygen saturation above 90%. Excessive oxygen concentrations can cause oxidative injury to tissues, so the goal is to minimize FiO2 while maintaining adequate oxygenation. Hyperoxia, particularly in post-arrest patients, can be detrimental.

PEEP Considerations

PEEP is essential for preventing alveolar collapse (atelectasis) and reducing the risk of atelectrauma. The optimal PEEP is typically set to the lowest level that prevents alveolar collapse. An initial PEEP of 5 cm H2O is commonly used, especially in patients with no significant oxygenation issues. For hypoxemic patients, PEEP should be adjusted in conjunction with FiO2 to maintain adequate oxygenation without exceeding a plateau pressure of 30 cm H2O. The use of PEEP is titrated based on oxygenation goals, and increasing PEEP beyond 15 cm H2O does not improve survival and may compromise hemodynamics.

Recruitment Maneuvers

Recruitment maneuvers temporarily increase airway pressure to open collapsed alveoli, and after successful recruitment, PEEP is increased to maintain this opening. Recruitment can be performed using higher ventilator settings or by using an Ambu bag with a PEEP valve.

Common protocols use a BiLevel mode with high PEEP (40 cm H2O) for up to 20 seconds, with the maneuver stopped if the patient experiences hypotension, hypoxemia, or arrhythmias. While recruitment may improve oxygenation and lung compliance in some cases, it has not been shown to consistently improve outcomes and can cause complications such as pneumothorax and hypotension.

Adjusting Mechanical Ventilation

Ventilation Changes
Mechanical ventilation settings should be adjusted regularly based on the patient's evolving condition. Changes in lung compliance, minute ventilation, and oxygenation demands necessitate periodic reassessment and adjustment. Blood gases should be measured 15-30 minutes after initial settings and after any changes to ensure the pH is in the normal range and tidal volume goals are met.

Adjusting to Maintain Normal pH

In general, increasing minute ventilation will lower CO2 levels, raising the pH. However, the effects of adjustments on CO2 clearance are not always predictable due to changes in dead space. Smaller tidal volumes can result in higher dead space and less effective CO2 clearance. It's important to balance the tidal volume and respiratory rate to avoid complications such as impaired CO2 clearance, especially in patients with obstructive lung diseases.

Tidal Volume Adjustment for ARDSNet Recommendations

In patients with ARDS, low tidal volumes of 6-7 mL/kg of ideal body weight are recommended. If the plateau pressure exceeds 30 cm H2O, tidal volumes may be further reduced. While this strategy may result in mild respiratory acidosis (permissive hypercapnia), it is generally well tolerated, provided the pH remains above 7.2. However, permissive hypercapnia is contraindicated in conditions like high intracranial pressure, myocardial instability, or severe pulmonary hypertension, as elevated $CO_2$ can worsen these conditions.

## Limitations and Considerations

Mechanical ventilation has limitations, especially in terms of minute ventilation and its impact on the patient's expiratory phase. These limitations are influenced by lung compliance, and adjustments may not always lead to predictable outcomes.

## Plateau Pressure Management
In both volume-targeted and pressure-targeted ventilation modes, plateau pressure should be kept below 30 cm $H_2O$. For volume-targeted ventilation, this requires intermittent measurement of plateau pressure, while in pressure-targeted ventilation, the plateau pressure is the sum of PEEP and the driving pressure. If plateau pressure exceeds 30 cm $H_2O$, further adjustments to tidal volume may be necessary.

Spontaneous Mode

In certain cases, such as during weaning trials or in patients who are awake and stable, the ventilator can be set to spontaneous mode, also known as pressure support ventilation (PSV). This mode allows the patient to take breaths as deep and as frequent as they wish, with a pressure support level set above PEEP. For weaning, typical settings are 5-8 cm H2O of pressure support. This mode is helpful for patients who are beginning to recover but still need support in maintaining adequate ventilation.

Right Heart Syndrome and Cor Pulmonale

The right heart has a limited capacity to manage increased afterload, responding primarily through dilation. Both the left and right ventricles are interdependent, sharing the same pericardial sac and septum. Any increase in the volume of one ventricle results in a corresponding decrease in space available for the other. As the right ventricle dilates, it can compress the left ventricle, reducing its diastolic size. This compression can impair left ventricular output, potentially leading to a drop in systemic blood pressure.

The perfusion of the right ventricle depends on the pressure gradient between its internal pressure and the systemic arterial pressure. As the right ventricle dilates and pulmonary pressures rise, typically due to left heart failure, hypoxemia, or acidosis, systemic pressures decrease. This combined reduction in systemic pressures and increase in pulmonary pressures exacerbates ischemia, creating a self-perpetuating cycle of deterioration.

Left Heart Afterload

The left heart pumps blood into the systemic vasculature, which is outside the chest. Consequently, its function is influenced by changes in intrathoracic pressure. Under normal circumstances, negative pressure during inhalation helps draw blood into the left heart, enhancing output. This is generally a minor impediment, easily compensated for by the heart.

However, during conditions like Acute Respiratory Distress Syndrome (ARDS) or upper airway obstructions (e.g., stridor), extreme fluctuations in intrathoracic pressure can cause a significant reduction in cardiac output and may contribute to left heart failure.

Conversely, positive pressure ventilation can relieve afterload in the left heart by compressing the thorax and increasing cardiac output, thus supporting left heart function in patients experiencing failure.

Post-Intubation Hypotension

The transition to mechanical ventilation is frequently accompanied by hemodynamic instability, reflecting the close interaction between the heart and lungs. Several factors contribute to this instability:

1. Changes in Adrenergic Tone and Drug Effects: Induction agents used for intubation can have direct hemodynamic effects, often reducing sympathetic tone and lowering blood pressure. Patients with elevated adrenergic tone before intubation are particularly susceptible to this effect. Additionally, some sedatives or induction drugs may be negatively inotropic or induce vasoplegia, further exacerbating hypotension.

2. Changes in Preload: Positive pressure ventilation impedes venous return to the right heart, which can be particularly problematic in hypovolemic patients. Reduced preload can further compromise right ventricular output.

3. Changes in Afterload: Patients with pre-existing right heart failure are at risk for increased pulmonary vascular pressure when positive pressure ventilation is initiated. This

sudden rise in pressure can overwhelm the right heart, causing a decrease in cardiac output.

4. Changes in Oxygenation and Ventilation: The administration of sedatives and paralytics during intubation leads to apnea, decreasing functional residual capacity (FRC) and precipitating rapid hypoxemia and hypercapnia. This is especially problematic in patients with low FRC, such as pregnant women or morbidly obese individuals, and can result in significant hemodynamic compromise.

Remedies for Post-Intubation Hemodynamic Issues

To address the potential hemodynamic instability following mechanical ventilation initiation, it is critical to anticipate and prepare for these challenges. Careful monitoring is essential immediately after intubation, ensuring the patient remains stable before any changes to their management are made.

Fluid Resuscitation: In cases of suspected hypovolemia (e.g., patients with inadequate oral intake, excessive diuresis, or gastrointestinal loss), fluid boluses should be administered promptly.

Vasopressors: Pressor agents should be prepared and available for use, especially if the patient is already hypotensive. If needed, starting vasopressors at a low rate or utilizing push-dose pressors can provide immediate support to maintain perfusion.

The goal is to stabilize the patient's hemodynamics promptly, ensuring that they remain supported throughout the intubation and ventilation process.

# Chapter Six
# Complications of Mechanical Ventilation

Mechanical ventilation, although lifesaving, is not without its complications, which can hinder or delay a patient's recovery. The following section discusses common complications, their underlying mechanisms, and strategies for minimizing these risks.

Ventilator-Induced Lung Injury (VILI)

Mechanical ventilation can cause direct damage to lung tissue with each breath delivered. The mechanical force involved in ventilating the lungs stretches and potentially tears delicate alveolar structures. While the goal is for the patient's condition to improve more rapidly than the damage caused by ventilation accumulates, this is not always the case. When the patient's pathology does not recover quickly enough, mechanical ventilation may no longer be beneficial, resulting in prolonged dependence on the ventilator.

The primary mechanism by which mechanical ventilation harms the lungs is through excessive pressure and stretch applied to the lung tissue. This damage can lead to alveolar rupture, leakage, and progressive respiratory failure, which may mimic Acute Respiratory Distress Syndrome (ARDS) after a period of mechanical ventilation.

Volutrauma

Volutrauma refers to lung injury caused by overdistention from excessive tidal volumes. This is especially problematic in conditions like ARDS, where areas of lung tissue become consolidated and non-ventilated. The remaining functional lung tissue may be overinflated by high-volume breaths. To minimize volutrauma, it's crucial to adhere to established protocols for tidal volume management, such as those recommended by ARDSnet. These protocols have been shown to reduce mortality and should be followed closely for patients with ARDS and other forms of mechanical ventilation.

Barotrauma

Barotrauma occurs when excessive pressure is applied to lung tissues, particularly through high transmural pressures. The transmural pressure is the difference between the pressure inside the lung and that outside. Low transmural pressure does not typically cause damage, even with high internal pressures, while high transmural pressure can lead to injury regardless of the internal pressure.

For example, in morbidly obese patients, high intrapulmonary pressures may be necessary to achieve ventilation, but the weight of the abdomen and chest counteracts this pressure, preventing lung injury. In contrast, patients with low intrapulmonary pressures but high negative pleural pressures can experience significant damage due to large trans-pulmonary pressure gradients. Barotrauma can result in pneumothoraces, pneumomediastinum, and subcutaneous emphysema.

To prevent barotrauma, it is crucial to manage plateau pressures (ideally under 30 cmH2O) and driving pressures (ideally under 15 cmH2O). While these measures are helpful, they do not account for the full effect of transmural pressure on lung tissue.

Atelectotrauma

Atelectotrauma is caused by the repeated collapse and reopening of alveoli during ventilation. This cyclic process leads to tissue damage, particularly in cases of non-compliant lungs. To reduce atelectrauma, strategies include maintaining alveolar stability by using appropriate positive end-expiratory pressure (PEEP) and limiting tidal volumes. The ideal PEEP can be determined by assessing the pressure-volume curve and targeting the lower inflection point, where lung compliance improves as previously collapsed alveoli reopen.

Ventilator-Associated Pneumonia (VAP)

VAP is a common and serious complication of mechanical ventilation. It is suspected when a patient on mechanical ventilation develops a new or worsening clinical condition, including respiratory distress, increased secretions, new imaging findings, and signs of infection such as fever or elevated white blood cell counts.

The diagnosis of VAP involves obtaining lower respiratory tract samples, such as an endotracheal aspirate, and blood cultures. Empiric antibiotic therapy should be guided by hospital antibiograms, considering the patient's history and potential exposure to resistant organisms.

Prevention Strategies for VAP:

Use non-invasive ventilation when appropriate.

Elevate the head of the bed to 30-45 degrees.

Incorporate subglottic drainage systems for endotracheal tubes.

Perform daily assessments for extubation readiness.

Implement oral care protocols, including chlorhexidine in certain settings.

Airway Injury and Endotracheal Tube Complications

The endotracheal tube, while essential for mechanical ventilation, can also contribute to patient harm. Complications can arise from both the intubation procedure and the prolonged presence of the tube.

Intubation-related Complications:

Damage to the teeth, mouth, and upper airway structures, especially in emergency intubation situations.

Pressure from the securing device (e.g., tape or tube holder) can cause skin breakdown and pressure ulcers.

Complications During Prolonged Intubation:

The endotracheal tube may cause pressure ulcers in the mouth, lips, or oropharynx, and it can lead to damage to the vocal cords or trachea, causing ischemia and potentially leading to tracheal stenosis or malacia.

The cuff, which seals the airway, can exert pressure on the tracheal walls, leading to ischemia, which may result in tracheal damage over time, particularly in patients with low blood pressure or high cuff pressures.

To prevent these complications, the following measures are recommended:

Carefully select the appropriate tube size, with general guidelines suggesting a 7.5 tube for women and an 8.0 tube for men.

Use minimal cuff pressures, monitored using a cuff manometer, and employ techniques such as "minimal occluding volume" or "minimal leak" to ensure safe cuff pressure.

Remove the endotracheal tube as soon as clinically feasible to reduce the risk of complications.

Weakness and Deconditioning

Mechanical ventilation can lead to significant muscle weakness, even after a relatively short period of use (as little as four days). This weakness, often associated with critical illness myopathy, is compounded by prolonged sedation and immobility. It can significantly prolong the patient's recovery time and is associated with increased long-term mortality.

Management Strategies:

Early mobilization and physical therapy, even in patients on mechanical ventilation, can reduce the duration of ventilation and improve outcomes.

Sedation and Delirium

Sedation is essential to prevent discomfort and agitation in mechanically ventilated patients. However, the use of sedatives can contribute to delirium, prolonging the need for mechanical ventilation and increasing the risk of complications. Protocols to minimize sedation should be in place, and patients should be regularly assessed for readiness to wean off sedation when possible.

## Gastric Ulcers and Bleeding

Critically ill patients on mechanical ventilation are at high risk for gastric ulcers due to the loss of the protective mucosal barrier. Stress ulcer prophylaxis, including the use of H2 blockers or proton pump inhibitors (PPIs), is recommended for patients ventilated for more than 48 hours. However, PPIs may increase the risk of Clostridium difficile infections, which must be considered when selecting prophylaxis strategies.

## Ileus and Constipation

Sedation, immobility, and poor perfusion contribute to a high incidence of ileus and constipation in mechanically ventilated patients. Early implementation of a bowel regimen and regular monitoring of bowel function are important, particularly for patients receiving paralytics or deep sedation.

Deep Vein Thrombosis (DVT) and Pulmonary Embolism (PE)

Due to prolonged sedation and immobility, mechanically ventilated patients are at increased risk for DVTs and pulmonary embolism, even with prophylactic measures in place. It is crucial to maintain a high index of suspicion for these conditions, especially in patients with risk factors such as malignancy or central venous lines.

Conclusion

The complications associated with mechanical ventilation, while often preventable or manageable, can significantly impact patient outcomes. Awareness and adherence to institutional protocols can help minimize these risks, ensuring that mechanical ventilation remains a life-saving intervention rather than a source of harm.

## Chapter Seven
## Discontinuing Mechanical Ventilation

In the intensive care unit (ICU), one of the primary responsibilities of the medical team is to determine when to discontinue mechanical ventilation. The decision to stop mechanical ventilation should begin to be considered as soon as it is initiated. Prolonged mechanical ventilation increases the likelihood of complications, such as ventilator-associated pneumonia (VAP), mechanical issues, and sedation-related problems. The longer a patient remains intubated, the greater the risk of these complications.

Complications of Mechanical Ventilation

Common complications of mechanical ventilation include ventilator-associated pneumonia, which occurs in approximately 1%

of intubated patients each day. The mortality rate for VAP can be as high as 20-50%. Other mechanical risks involve accidental dislodgement of the tube, or damage to the laryngeal and tracheal structures. Additionally, patients who are sedated and immobile are at risk of muscle deconditioning and other issues. Dyssynchrony between the patient and ventilator, often due to oversedation, can lead to lung injury and respiratory muscle damage. Therefore, ICU management aims to wean patients off the ventilator as soon as it is clinically appropriate.

Risks of Premature Extubation

Premature extubation can have serious consequences. If extubation fails, the patient may experience airway loss, hypoxemia, and hemodynamic instability. Failed extubation is linked to higher mortality rates, increased risk of nosocomial pneumonia, prolonged ICU stays, and a significant increase in hospital costs—up to $35,000. Thus, careful assessment is crucial before discontinuing mechanical ventilation.

Criteria for Discontinuation of Mechanical Ventilation

To determine when a patient is ready for extubation, several criteria must be met:

The underlying cause of respiratory failure must be resolved.

The patient must demonstrate adequate oxygenation, typically with a fraction of inspired oxygen ($FiO_2$) of no more than 0.4 and a positive end-expiratory pressure (PEEP) of no more than 5 cm $H_2O$.

The patient should be hemodynamically stable.

The patient must be capable of initiating inspiratory effort and protecting their airway.

## Assessing Readiness for Extubation

Clinical judgment alone is not sufficient to determine readiness for extubation. It must be supplemented by objective clinical parameters, with the most reliable data coming from spontaneous breathing trials (SBT). These trials evaluate whether the patient can maintain adequate ventilation and oxygenation without the support of the ventilator.

## Spontaneous Breathing Trials (SBT)

The purpose of an SBT is to assess the patient's ability to breathe independently. During the trial, ventilatory support is reduced to allow the patient to perform the work of breathing. There are various SBT techniques, with the most common being the pressure support trial. In this method, the patient is placed on spontaneous mode with a low pressure support (5-8 cm H2O). This setup minimizes the resistance of the endotracheal tube and allows for monitoring of the patient's respiratory rate and breath depth.

Another method is the T-piece trial, where the patient is detached from the ventilator and allowed to breathe through a circuit without support.

Advantages and Disadvantages of SBT Techniques

The pressure support trial is often preferred as it has been shown to reduce the duration of mechanical ventilation. The patient remains attached to the ventilator, which ensures safety through alarms and a backup rate. The T-piece trial, while less commonly used, may be employed when there is concern that minimal PEEP may be necessary to prevent respiratory failure after extubation.

Failure of the Spontaneous Breathing Trial

A failed SBT is indicated by signs of patient fatigue, including rapid shallow breathing, reduced tidal volumes, and increased respiratory rates. The rapid shallow breathing index (RSBI), which is the ratio of respiratory rate to tidal volume (in liters), is often used to quantify this response. An RSBI greater than 105 is typically considered indicative of failure. While the RSBI is good at predicting extubation failure, it is less effective at predicting success. Factors such as auto-PEEP in COPD patients or neurologically impaired patients may skew the results. Other signs of failure include significant hypertension (>180 mmHg), hypotension (<90 mmHg), tachycardia, anxiety, and diaphoresis.

Management of Failed SBTs

When an SBT fails, it is important to identify the cause, which may include insufficient recovery from the primary illness or emerging complications such as volume overload, ventilator-associated pneumonia, or oversedation. In most cases, the failed trial should not be repeated within 24 hours, as muscle fatigue and other factors require time to recover. During this period, full ventilatory support is typically continued to assist with weaning.

Successful Spontaneous Breathing Trial

If a patient successfully completes an SBT without signs of fatigue or significant derangements in oxygenation, extubation should be considered. However, passing the SBT does not guarantee successful extubation, as other factors, such as airway protection and patency, must also be evaluated.

Airway Protection and Patency

Airway protection is essential for a successful extubation. The patient must be alert and able to clear secretions effectively. This is typically assessed by observing the patient's responsiveness and ability to protect the airway from aspiration. A weak cough or difficulty clearing secretions may indicate inadequate airway protection, even if the patient is alert.

For patients at risk of airway compromise, such as those with traumatic intubation or prolonged ventilation, a "leak test" can assess airway patency. This test involves deflating the endotracheal balloon and measuring the amount of gas leakage. Significant leakage may suggest sufficient airway patency, while the absence of leakage may indicate a risk of airway collapse upon extubation. In such cases, steroid trials may help manage upper airway edema.

Extubation Procedure

Once all criteria are met—successful SBT, adequate airway protection, and patency—extubation can proceed. The endotracheal tube is removed, and the patient is typically provided with supplemental humidified oxygen. Close monitoring for signs of stridor or respiratory distress is essential. Medication doses, particularly sedatives, should be adjusted accordingly.

## Extubation Failure

Even after a successful weaning trial, extubation may still fail. Post-extubation complications such as muscle deconditioning, poor nutrition, airway edema, or sedative effects can contribute to failure. Non-invasive ventilation (NIV) may be useful to support the patient during this critical period, particularly for those at high risk for respiratory failure, such as patients with COPD or those at risk of pulmonary edema.

## Prolonged Mechanical Ventilation

Some patients experience prolonged dependence on mechanical ventilation, which occurs in 1-5% of cases. This can be due to the primary illness or the complications of ventilation itself, such as weakness, ventilator-associated pneumonia, and delirium. The decision to continue or discontinue mechanical ventilation depends on the patient's progress and response to treatment.

## Tracheostomy in Prolonged Ventilation

For patients who are expected to require long-term ventilation, a tracheostomy may be considered. This procedure offers a more comfortable interface with the ventilator, reducing sedation requirements and facilitating easier suctioning. However, it carries risks, including bleeding, infection, and damage to the tracheal structures. The timing of a tracheostomy remains a debated issue, but it is typically considered after about 10 days of mechanical ventilation, especially in patients with neurologic conditions or neuromuscular diseases that result in slow recovery.

In patients who are not improving and are likely to require long-term ventilatory support, a tracheostomy may be necessary to improve comfort and quality of life. This decision should be made carefully, balancing the risks and benefits of the procedure.

## Chapter Eight
## Ventilation in Specialized Scenarios

Managing mechanical ventilation effectively in particular scenarios requires understanding the unique physiological and pathological considerations of each condition. Below is a focused discussion on the ventilation strategies for key clinical scenarios.

Acute Respiratory Distress Syndrome (ARDS)

ARDS is a clinical syndrome characterized by acute lung injury (typically within a week of onset), diffuse pulmonary infiltrates, and severe oxygenation impairment that is not attributable to cardiac-related pulmonary edema.

Etiology and Pathophysiology

ARDS arises from either direct pulmonary insults (e.g., pneumonia, inhalation injuries) or systemic inflammatory processes (e.g., pancreatitis, sepsis). The hallmark pathological feature is diffuse alveolar damage, resulting in alveolar consolidation and intrapulmonary shunting.

Severity Classification

The severity of ARDS is determined by the ratio of arterial oxygen partial pressure (PaO2) to the fraction of inspired oxygen (FiO2), termed the P/F ratio:

Mild: P/F ratio < 300

Moderate: P/F ratio < 200

Severe: P/F ratio < 100

Management Principles

While no specific pharmacological cure exists, managing ARDS involves treating the underlying cause and supporting the lungs to repair over time. Ventilation strategies are aimed at optimizing oxygenation while minimizing ventilator-induced lung injury.

Low Tidal Volume Ventilation: Adhering to ARDSNet protocols (6 mL/kg predicted body weight) minimizes barotrauma and volutrauma. Overdistention of the "baby lung" (the remaining ventilated lung) must be avoided to prevent further injury.

Plateau Pressure Limits: Maintaining plateau pressures ≤30 cm $H_2O$ reduces mechanical stress on alveoli.

Refractory Hypoxemia

Patients with ARDS and oxygenation unresponsive to basic interventions (e.g., PEEP < 10 cm $H_2O$ and $FiO_2$ < 60%) require advanced management strategies.

## Optimizing Ventilation-Perfusion (V/Q) Matching

Techniques to improve oxygenation include increasing mean airway pressure, using recruitment maneuvers, and fine-tuning PEEP levels:

PEEP Adjustments: Incremental increases can recruit collapsed alveoli but should be monitored closely to avoid hemodynamic compromise or increased dead space. Capnometry may aid in real-time adjustments.

Inspiratory Time Prolongation: Extending inspiratory time (or inverse ratio ventilation) can enhance alveolar recruitment and oxygenation.

## Sedation and Paralysis

Sedation: Agitation and dyssynchrony significantly increase oxygen demand. Adequate sedation with anxiolytics and analgesics reduces oxygen consumption.

Neuromuscular Blockade: Short-term use (≤48 hours) of paralytics may improve oxygenation and survival in select cases, although prolonged use risks muscle weakness.

Prone Positioning

Prone positioning improves oxygenation by redistributing ventilation and perfusion, enhancing dependent lung recruitment, and alleviating compression on caudal lung regions from the heart and abdominal organs. Early implementation in severe ARDS has demonstrated survival benefits.

Inhaled Vasodilators

Inhaled agents like nitric oxide or epoprostenol can temporarily improve oxygenation by redistributing pulmonary blood flow to better-ventilated regions. However, these therapies lack proven survival benefits and are primarily a bridge to definitive care, such as ECMO.

## Extracorporeal Membrane Oxygenation (ECMO)

For patients with refractory hypoxemia despite optimized conventional ventilation, ECMO offers a life-saving option.

### Indications and Mechanism

Suitable for reversible causes of respiratory failure (e.g., ARDS from infection).

Large catheters remove venous blood, oxygenate it extracorporeally, and return it to the arterial system.

Challenges and Considerations

Complications: ECMO is associated with bleeding, thrombosis, infection, and mechanical failure of the circuit.

Finite Duration: Prolonged ECMO risk complications, necessitating recovery or transition (e.g., lung transplant) within a limited timeframe.

Right Heart Stress and Cor Pulmonale

In ARDS, elevated pulmonary pressures from hypoxemia, hypercapnia, and ventilatory interventions strain the right ventricle (RV), potentially leading to cor pulmonale—a marker of poor prognosis.

## Management

Strategies to minimize RV stress include:

Reducing oxygen demand.

Optimizing volume status to prevent RV overload.

Avoiding excessive PEEP, which may compromise cardiac output.

## Pregnancy and Respiratory Changes

### Physiological Adjustments

Pregnancy induces significant respiratory system changes, primarily due to the gravid uterus and the increased metabolic demands of the growing fetus. Functional residual capacity (FRC) decreases, chest wall compliance is reduced, and oxygen consumption rises. These adaptations make pregnant patients more susceptible to cardiopulmonary disturbances, potentially necessitating mechanical ventilation even in this otherwise resilient demographic.

Normal pregnancy physiology leads to increased tidal volume and mild respiratory alkalosis ($pCO_2$: 27–34 mmHg), driven by progesterone's stimulatory effect. The reduction in FRC and heightened oxygen utilization predispose patients to rapid desaturation during anesthesia induction.

Airway Challenges and Risk Mitigation
Pregnant patients are considered difficult airway cases due to anatomical and physiological changes, such as mucosal edema, capillary engorgement, and reduced lower esophageal tone. Smaller endotracheal tubes are often required. Gastric emptying delays and increased intra-abdominal pressure elevate aspiration risk. If non-invasive ventilation is used, patients must exhibit intact protective airway reflexes and stable hemodynamics. However, this modality should be reserved for reversible causes of

respiratory failure, with close monitoring due to aspiration risks.

Mechanical Ventilation Goals
For mechanically ventilated pregnant patients, the primary objectives are to maintain a PaO$_2$ of approximately 70 mmHg and oxygen saturation above 95%. Permissive hypercapnia is avoided due to its potential to cause fetal acidosis, while respiratory alkalosis (pH >7.48) should also be prevented to avoid uterine artery constriction. Ventilator settings should balance maternal and fetal safety, with ARDSNet-recommended plateau pressure targets ensuring lung protection.

Abnormal Breathing Patterns

Cheyne-Stokes Respiration
This cyclic breathing pattern features waxing and waning respiratory depth, interspersed with apnea. Its recognition is essential to avoid inappropriate ventilator adjustments, which may exacerbate dyssynchrony. During the crescendo

phase, pressure-targeted modes minimize flow dyssynchrony. Apnea alarms can be adjusted during weaning trials to reduce disruptions.

### Kussmaul Breathing

Deep, rapid breathing is characteristic of metabolic acidosis states like diabetic ketoacidosis (DKA). Synchronizing ventilator settings with this breathing pattern is critical to prevent hemodynamic compromise. Temporary adjustments, such as low-pressure support modes, can alleviate dyssynchrony while the underlying acidosis is corrected.

## Specialized Ventilation Scenarios

### ECMO Support

Extracorporeal membrane oxygenation (ECMO) offers an alternative for patients with refractory cardiogenic shock or hypoxemia, bypassing the need for high ventilator pressures. Once on ECMO, ventilatory support is minimized to prevent lung injury, with settings such as low pressure support (PEEP 5–10 cm $H_2O$). Extubation may be considered if the patient is alert with intact airway reflexes.

Pneumothorax and Bronchopleural Fistulas
Patients with air leaks require ventilator adjustments to minimize exacerbation. Low-volume, minimal-pressure strategies reduce the risk of further damage. Avoiding auto-cycling is crucial, as this can trigger respiratory alkalosis.

Right Heart Failure and Pulmonary Hypertension
Initiating mechanical ventilation in these patients carries a high risk of hemodynamic collapse due to increased pulmonary vascular resistance. Vasopressors should be readily available, and strategies to mitigate pulmonary stress are essential.

## Morbid Obesity and Respiratory Management

Morbidly obese patients share physiological challenges with pregnancy, including reduced FRC and increased oxygen demand. Ventilation strategies should focus on ideal body weight for tidal volume calculations. Higher PEEP and plateau pressures may be necessary, though these must be carefully titrated. Supine positioning exacerbates autoPEEP risks, so strategies to optimize ventilation in this population are essential.

## References

1. Bateman, N. T., & Leach, R. M. (1998). Acute oxygen therapy. BMJ: British Medical Journal, 317(7161), 798–801. https://doi.org/10.1136/bmj.317.7161.798.

2. Blanch, L., Villagra, A., Sales, B., Montanya, J., Lucangelo, U., Luján, M., García-Esquirol, O., et al. (2015). Associations between ventilation asynchronies and patient mortality. Intensive Care Medicine, 41(4), 633–641. https://doi.org/10.1007/s00134-015-3692-6.

3. Bone, R. C., & Burch, S. G. (1991). Management strategies for status . Annals of Allergy, 67(5), 461–469.

4. Cavalcanti, A. B., Suzumura, É. A., Laranjeira, L. N., Paisani, D. M., Damiani, L. P., Guimarães, H. P., Romano, E. R., et al. (2017). Comparing lung recruitment and PEEP titration

strategies with low PEEP for acute respiratory distress syndrome. JAMA, 318(14), 1335–1345. https://doi.org/10.1001/jama.2017.14171.

5. Chaudhuri, A., & Behan, P. O. (2009). Clinical considerations in myasthenic crisis. QJM: An International Journal of Medicine, 102(2), 97–107. https://doi.org/10.1093/qjmed/hcn152.

6. Cook, D. J., Walter, S. D., Cook, R. J., Griffith, L. E., Guyatt, G. H., Leasa, D., Jaeschke, R. Z., & Brun-Buisson, C. (1998). Ventilator-associated pneumonia incidence and contributing factors. Annals of Internal Medicine, 129(6), 433–440. https://doi.org/10.7326/0003-4819-129-6-199809150-00002.

7. Disselkamp, M., Adkins, D., Pandey, S., & Coz Yataco, A. O. (2018). Mechanically ventilating patients with right ventricular failure: A physiological perspective. Annals of the American Thoracic Society, 15(3), 383–389.

https://doi.org/10.1513/AnnalsATS.201707-533 CC.

8. Duan, J., Han, X., Bai, L., Zhou, L., & Huang, S. (2017). Predicting noninvasive ventilation failure in hypoxemic patients using respiratory and metabolic markers. Intensive Care Medicine, 43(2), 192–199. https://doi.org/10.1007/s00134-016-4601-3.

9. Esteban, A., Anzueto, A., Alia, I., et al. (2000). Patterns of mechanical ventilation in ICU settings: An international review. American Journal of Respiratory and Critical Care Medicine, 151, 1450–1458.

10. Girardis, M., Busani, S., Damiani, E., Donati, A., Rinaldi, L., Marudi, A., Morelli, A., Antonelli, M., & Singer, M. (2016). Impact of conservative versus conventional oxygen therapy on ICU mortality: Findings from the Oxygen-ICU randomized trial. JAMA, 316(15), 1583–1589.
https://doi.org/10.1001/jama.2016.11993.

11. ICU-ROX Investigators, & Australian and New Zealand Intensive Care Society Clinical Trials Group, Mackle, D., Bellomo, R., Bailey, M., Beasley, R., Deane, A., Eastwood, G., et al. (2020). Conservative oxygen strategies during mechanical ventilation in the ICU. New England Journal of Medicine, 382(11), 989–998. https://doi.org/10.1056/NEJMoa1903297.

12. Kalil, A. C., Metersky, M. L., Klompas, M., Muscedere, J., Sweeney, D. A., Palmer, L. B., Napolitano, L. M., et al. (2016). Guidelines for managing hospital-acquired and ventilator-associated pneumonia. Clinical Infectious Diseases, 63(5), e61–111. https://doi.org/10.1093/cid/ciw353.

13. Kallet, R. H., Alonso, J. A., Luce, J. M., & Matthay, M. A. (1999). Worsened pulmonary edema during low-tidal-volume, lung-protective ventilation strategies. Chest, 116(6), 1826–1832. https://doi.org/10.1378/chest.116.6.1826.

14. Klompas, M., Branson, R., Eichenwald, E. C., Greene, L. R., Howell, M. D., Lee, G., Magill, S. S., et al. (2014). Strategies to minimize ventilator-associated pneumonia in acute care settings. Infection Control and Hospital Epidemiology, 35(8), 915–936. https://doi.org/10.1086/677144.

15. Laghi, F., & Goyal, A. (2012). Auto-PEEP implications in respiratory failure. Minerva Anestesiologica, 78(2), 201–221.

16. Laghi, F., Karamchandani, K., & Tobin, M. J. (1999). Ventilator settings and their influence on respiratory frequency during mechanical support. American Journal of Respiratory and Critical Care Medicine, 160(5 Pt 1), 1766–1770. https://doi.org/10.1164/ajrccm.160.5.9810086.

17. Leonhard, S. E., Mandarakas, M. R., Gondim, F. A. A., Bateman, K., Ferreira, M. L. B., Cornblath, D. R., van Doorn, P. A., et al. (2019). Key steps for diagnosing and managing Guillain-Barré Syndrome. Nature Reviews

Neurology, 15(11), 671–683. https://doi.org/10.1038/s41582-019-0250-9.

## Glossary

**Acute Respiratory Distress Syndrome (ARDS):** A severe form of lung injury characterized by diffuse alveolar damage, leading to respiratory failure and requiring mechanical ventilation.

**Barotrauma**: Lung injury caused by excessive pressure during mechanical ventilation, potentially leading to alveolar rupture and air leaks.

**Chronic Obstructive Pulmonary Disease (COPD):** A chronic lung disease involving airflow obstruction, often managed with specific ventilation strategies to reduce air trapping and hyperinflation.

**Extracorporeal Membrane Oxygenation (ECMO):** A life-support technique that uses an external device to oxygenate and remove carbon dioxide from the blood in cases of severe respiratory failure.

**FiO2 (Fraction of Inspired Oxygen):** The concentration of oxygen delivered to the patient via the ventilator, typically adjusted based on oxygenation needs.

**High-Frequency Oscillatory Ventilation (HFOV):** An advanced ventilation mode using rapid, small-volume breaths to minimize lung injury while ensuring gas exchange.

**Neuromuscular Disorders**: Conditions affecting the nerves and muscles, often requiring ventilatory support due to weakened respiratory muscles.

**Noninvasive Ventilation (NIV):** A ventilation method using masks or other interfaces to support breathing without invasive airway devices like endotracheal tubes.

**PEEP (Positive End-Expiratory Pressure):** A ventilatory setting that maintains airway pressure at the end of exhalation to prevent alveolar collapse and improve oxygenation.

**Tidal Volume (VT):** The amount of air delivered to the lungs with each ventilator breath, typically calculated based on the patient's ideal body weight.

**Ventilator-Associated Pneumonia (VAP):** A lung infection occurring in mechanically ventilated patients, often linked to prolonged intubation and inadequate hygiene measures.

**Volutrauma**: Lung injury resulting from overdistension of alveoli due to high tidal volumes during mechanical ventilation.

**Waveforms**: Graphical representations of ventilatory parameters, including pressure, flow, and volume, used for monitoring and troubleshooting ventilator performance.

**Weaning**: The gradual process of reducing ventilatory support to allow the patient to resume spontaneous breathing.

www.ingramcontent.com/pod-product-compliance
Lightning Source LLC
Chambersburg PA
CBHW071023240526
45469CB00006BD/2053